THE DRCOG EXAMINATION
A Structured Approach

THE DRCOG EXAMINATION
A Structured Approach

Stuart Mellor MB ChB MRCOG
Consultant Obstetrician and Gynaecologist
Macclesfield District General Hospital, Cheshire.
Diploma Examiner of the Royal College of Obstetricians and Gynaecologists.

Michael Read MD FRCS MRCOG FRACOG
Consultant Obstetrician and Gynaecologist, Gloucester.
Diploma Examiner of the Royal College of Obstetricians and Gynaecologists.

Stuart Bootle BSc(Hons) MB ChB DRCOG MRCGP
General Practitioner.

John Sandars MB ChB(Hons) MRCP MRCGP
Trainer in General Practice, Stockport.
Examiner, Royal College of General Practitioners.

© 1990 PASTEST SERVICE
Cranford Lodge, Bexton Road
Knutsford, Cheshire WA16 0ED
Telephone: 0565–755226

First published 1990
Reprinted 1990
Reprinted 1992

British Library Cataloguing in Publication Data

The DRCOG examination.
  1. Gynaecology & Obstetrics
  I. Mellor, Stuart
  618

ISBN 0 906896 614

Text prepared by Turner Associates, Knutsford, Cheshire.
Typeset by Speedset Ltd, Ellesmere Port.
Printed by Billing and Sons Ltd, Worcester.

CONTENTS

INTRODUCTION

A candidate about to sit the DRCOG examination needs to do a certain amount of work as one cannot reasonably expect to pass without having grasped the basic facts and principles of the subject.

However, having acquired this knowledge you then need to convince the examiners that you are sufficiently competent and proficient in obstetrics and gynaecology not to be a danger to your patients and are therefore worthy of passing the exam. The way in which the required information is presented, whether in a written paper, a clinical or in an oral examination can significantly influence the examiners, as they can only base their assessment on the information presented to them.

There are certain ways of presenting answers to best advantage, this is the art of passing exams and is the basis of this book.

The DRCOG examination is in three parts:

a)   The Written Paper: essay questions
                            multiple choice questions
b)   The Clinical Examination
c)   The Oral Examination

The way in which candidates revise for examinations varies enormously but by the time you are preparing for the diploma you should have found the method best suited to you.

As long as you cover the full syllabus in an unhurried manner, the precise method used is not important. However, last minute cramming, although surprisingly popular, is not to be recommended particularly in the diploma which is very practical in its orientation.

In this book we take each section in turn.

College Entry Requirements

The College awards the Diploma to registered Medical Practitioners who have had appropriate postgraduate training and who satisfy the examiners at the time of the examination. The potential examinee must:

a) be a fully registered Medical Practitioner, having completed 12 months in appointments acceptable for preregistration purposes (i.e. 'house jobs')

b) have held a post-registration appointment for 6 consecutive months, specifically recognised by the college, in obstetrics and gynaecology being resident on duty. Proof of this is required from the consultant in charge (e.g. VTR-2 form)

c) have adequate family planning training
        either – hold a Joint Committee on Contraception certificate
        or – have attended 8 family planning clinics and be competent at IUCD fitting (i.e. awaiting the certificate)
A green form will be sent with the application documents, on which these 8 sessions should be detailed. It will need to be signed by the instructing doctor. If you hold the JCC certificate, a copy will usually suffice

d) pay a fee (remember this is tax deductable and therefore worth declaring on your tax form)

e) complete an application form.

Full details and forms are available from:

The Examination Secretary
Royal College of Obstetricians & Gynaecologists
27 Sussex Place
London NW1 4RG
Tel: 01 262 5425

It is worth applying early in order to complete the various forms, especially the family planning forms, before the closing date.

The Examination Day

Having passed a usually troubled and seemingly endless night, it is at last time to get up. Give yourself plenty of time.

It is important that you are comfortable during the exam. Wear whatever clothing you feel most comfortable in, there is no need for 'exam attire' for the written paper.

If you are taking the exam in a distant centre make sure you book your accommodation well in advance. It is not a good idea to travel a long distance on the day of the exam as hold ups can and do occur which add unnecessary stress to the already anxious candidate. Remember that no allowance is made for late arrival.

After arriving at the place where you are staying make sure you know the way to the examination centre. If you have not been there before it can be very helpful to make the journey beforehand so that you then have an idea of the distance involved and the time it is likely to take. Be sure to allow extra time for rush hour travel.

Pre-examination tension builds up however well prepared you are, so try to occupy your mind with non-related topics. If travelling by rail you will find that a novel passes the time admirably and prevents brooding. Never take textbooks, it is far too late for them to do any good; they may well cause confusion and add to your anxiety.

Check that you have all the documentation you need to be admitted to the exam and take equipment with you for the clinicals. Leave in plenty of time to allow for unexpected delays. Aim to arrive at the centre 15–20 minutes before the exam starts, if you arrive too early the anxious chatter and cross questioning between the other candidates can have an unnerving effect.

For the written examination you will be admitted to the examination room 10–15 minutes before the examination is due to start. Leave coats, briefcases etc where indicated by the invigilators. Take your correct seat. There will be a card on the desk with your number on it which corresponds to the number on your admission card.

Do nothing more until instructed by the invigilator. Attempts to label books etc are pointless as time is allowed for this and if done incorrectly causes inconvenience to you and the invigilators. The person in charge will give full instructions about labelling attendance cards, answer books etc and on how the questions should be answered (all questions; separate books for each question; one side of each page etc). Listen carefully and if anything is unclear raise your hand and an invigilator will come to you to resolve your query.

The multiple choice paper will be first. Read the instructions printed on the paper carefully. On the front cover you must print your full name in the boxes provided and add your signature in the marked space. Your candidate number should be written in the four squares provided.

After the multiple choice paper of one and a quarter hours there will be a fifteen minute break whilst the papers are collected and essay questions distributed. There are two compulsory questions to be answered in one and a half hours and each question must be answered in a separate book.

Conclusion

Most candidates who fail, fail themselves. Errors of commission are much more common than errors of omission.

Our apologies in advance for any ambiguities that may have crept into the text or for any omissions that we should have covered however it is hoped that these hints will help you to avoid most pitfalls and will add a little extra 'finish' to your performance.

1. A DRCOG REVISION CHECKLIST

Preparation for the DRCOG examination can follow a structured approach using guidelines offered by the college at the time of application. It is hoped that reference to a 'checklist' of topics will ensure that the candidate covers all areas of the specialty. The potential examinee needs to keep up-to-date with recent advances in the field of obstetrics and gynaecology as the orals draw near. The following is offered as a checklist with boxes that you can tick as you complete your revision in each area.

OBSTETRICS:

☐ History taking
☐ Examination of abdomen in pregnancy
☐ Perinatal mortality figures and causes
☐ Maternal mortality figures and causes
☐ Preconception evaluation and counselling
☐ The diagnosis of pregnancy
☐ Antenatal care
    Role of the GP/Midwife/Primary Health Care Team
    Booking routines
    Criteria for GP care versus hospital care
    Prenatal diagnosis of abnormality
        AFP
        Triple hormone assay
        Amniocentesis
        Ultrasound
        Chorionic villus biopsy
        Fetoscopy

☐ Common minor problems in pregnancy
☐ Common major problems in pregnancy
    Placental insufficiency
    IUGR
    Pre-eclampsia and hypertensive disease
    Diabetes
    Thyroid problems
    Anaemia
    Urinary tract infections
    Abdominal pain

Heart disease
Rhesus disease
Antepartum haemorrhage
Hydatidiform mole
Hyperemesis
Malpresentations – Breech
               – Unstable lie
               – Transverse lie
Multiple pregnancy
Hydramnios
Fetal infection in pregnancy
  (TORCH)
Preterm labour
Premature rupture of membranes
Prolonged pregnancy and post maturity

☐ Intrapartum care
Home deliveries versus hospital deliveries
Diagnosis of labour
Physiology of normal labour
Mechanisms and management of normal labour
Documentation/partograms
Induction of labour - criteria/methods
Bishops score
1st Stage
    Intrapartum monitoring – CTG
                      – Scalp pH
    Pain relief
    Epidural anaesthesia
    Delay and management
    Bleeding and management
2nd Stage
    Definition of Delay
    Instrumental deliveries
    Assisted breech delivery
    Concept of fetal distress
    Episiotomy and lacerations
    Caesarean section
    Shoulder dystocia
    Twin delivery
3rd Stage
    Active management
    Concept of oxytocic (syntometrine)
    Postpartum haemorrhage

Bonding
Communication with mother and family

☐ Postnatal care
Routine examination of newborn
Resuscitation of newborn/Apgar scoring
Common abnormalities of the baby
Jaundice
Birth trauma
Care and feeding of the newborn
RDS
Diabetes and its risks
Low birth weight babies
Preterm babies

Physiology of puerperium
Breast feeding
Puerperal fever
Puerperal depression
Contraceptive advice
Rubella vaccination
Anti-D vaccination
The 6-week check
GP claim forms FP1001, FP1002
          FP24 and 24A

GYNAECOLOGY:

☐ History taking
☐ Examination of abdomen and pelvis
☐ Health education and preventative screening for women
☐ Physiology of menstrual cycle
☐ Congenital abnormalities
☐ Psychosexual counselling principles
☐ Menstrual problems
Amenorrhoea
Menorrhagia
Dysmenorrhoea
Premenstrual syndrome

☐ Puberty
☐ The menopause/Hormone Replacement Therapy (HRT)

- [ ] Pregnancy related problems
    - Abortion and habitual abortion
    - Ectopic pregnancy
- [ ] Infertility (including IVF and GIFT)
- [ ] Neoplasia
    - Breast
    - Uterine
    - Ovarian
    - Vaginal
    - Vulval
    - Cervical
- [ ] Cervical intra-epithelial neoplasia and cervical smears
- [ ] Colposcopy techniques
- [ ] Pelvic inflammatory disease
- [ ] Sexually transmitted disease (including AIDS)
- [ ] Vaginal infections and discharge
- [ ] Vulval dystrophy
- [ ] Fibroids
- [ ] Endometriosis
- [ ] Prolapse
- [ ] Urinary tract problems in women
    - Incontinence – stress
                         – urge
    - Urodynamic studies
    - Infections
- [ ] Common gynaecological operations

FAMILY PLANNING

- [ ] Failure rates, acceptability and motivation
- [ ] Natural methods
- [ ] Barrier methods: sheath/caps and diaphragms
- [ ] Spermicides
- [ ] Hormonal methods
    - Combined pill
    - Mini-pill
    - Injectables
    - Post-coital contraception
- [ ] IUCD
- [ ] Sterilisation
- [ ] Terminations
- [ ] Recent advances
    - 'female condom'

LHRH analogues
Male pill
☐ GP protocol including claim forms (FP1001, FP1002, FP1003)
☐ Family planning clinics

READING AND REFERENCE BOOKLIST

Brown, R. J. K. & Valman H. B. Practical Neonatal Paediatrics. 4th ed. 1979 Blackwell Scientific.

Chamberlain, G. **Lecture Notes on Gynaecology.** 6th ed. 1988. Blackwell Scientific.

Chamberlain, G. **Lecture Notes on Obstetrics.** 5th ed. 1984. Blackwell Scientific.

Chamberlain, G. & Dewhurst, J. **A Practice of Obstetrics and Gynaecology: A Primer for the DRCOG.** 2nd ed. 1984. Churchill Livingstone.

Clayton, S. G. **Obstetrics by Ten Teachers. Gynaecology by Ten Teachers.** 14th ed. 1985. Edward Arnold.

Kaye, P. **Notes for the DRCOG.** 2nd ed. 1988. Churchill Livingstone.

McPherson, A. & Anderson, A. **Women's Problems in General Practice.** 2nd ed. 1988. Oxford University Press.

Read, M. D. & Mellor, S. **Obstetrics in Outline.** 1985. Wiley

Read, M. D. & Mellor, S. **Guidelines to Gynaecology.** 1982. Blackwell Scientific.

Stirrat, G. M. **Aids to Obstetrics & Gynaecology.** 2nd ed. 1987. Churchill Livingstone.

Studd, J. et al. **Self-Assessment in Obstetrics and Gynaecology.** 1983. Blackwell Scientific.

Tindall, V. R. **MCQ Tutor Basic Sciences in Obstetrics and Gynaecology.** 1987. Heinemann.

Tindall, V. R. Martin, R. H. & Burslem, R. W. **Preparation and Advice for the MRCOG.** 1989. Churchill Livingstone.

Journals
Drugs and Therapeutics Bulletin
British National Formulary (BNF)
British Journal of Sexual Medicine
Journal of the Royal College of General Practitioners
British Medical Journal

2. THE WRITTEN EXAMINATION

THE MULTIPLE CHOICE QUESTION PAPER

The introduction of a Multiple Choice Question (MCQ) paper is a new aspect of the DRCOG examination.

Multiple Choice Questions are the most consistent, reproducible and internally reliable method we have of testing re-call of factual knowledge. Yet there is evidence that they are able to test more than simple factual re-call; reasoning ability and understanding of basic facts, principles and concepts can also be assessed. A good MCQ paper will discriminate accurately between candidates on the basis of their knowledge of the topics being tested. It must be emphasised that the most important function of an MCQ paper of the type used in the DRCOG, is to rank candidates accurately and fairly according to their performance in that paper. Accurate ranking is the key phrase; this means that all MCQ examinations of this type are in a sense competitive.

The MCQ paper consists of 40 multiple choice questions in book form and will include a broad spectrum of questions in obstetrics, gynaecology, family planning, paediatrics and associated subjects

Examination Technique

The safest way to pass the DRCOG is to know the answers to all of the questions, but it is equally important to be able to transfer this knowledge accurately onto the answer sheet. All too often, candidates suffer through an inability to organise their time, through failure to read the instructions carefully or through failure to read and understand the questions. First of all you must allocate your time with care. There are 40 questions to complete in 1¼ hours; this means under 2 minutes per question. Make sure that you are getting through the exam at least at this pace or if possible, a little quicker, thus allowing time at the end for revision and a re-think on some of the items that you have deferred.

It may be helpful for you to read through the whole paper first in order to get a feel for the total contents. Then you can go through the paper answering all the questions that you are sure of, i.e. immediate recall of information. Lastly go through the paper again slowly, answering all the questions that you can.

You must read the question (both stem and items) carefully. You should be quite clear that you know what you are being asked to do. Once you know this, you should indicate your responses by marking the paper boldly, correctly and clearly. Take great care not to mark the wrong boxes and think very carefully before making a mark on the computer answer sheet. Regard each item as being independent of every other item – each refers to a specific quantum of knowledge. The item (or the stem and the item taken together) make up a statement. You are required to indicate whether you regard this statement as 'True' or 'False' and if you do not know the answer then you *must* black out the 'Don't Know' box.

Marking your answer sheets

The answer sheet will be read by an automatic document reader, which transfers the information it reads to a computer. It must therefore be filled out in accordance with the instructions. A sample of the answer sheet, together with the instructions is available from the Royal College. Study these instructions carefully, well before the exams, the invigilators will also draw your attention to them at the time of the examination. You must first fill in your name on the answer sheet and then fill in your examination number. It is critical that this is filled in correctly with the 2B pencil provided.

As you go through the questions, you can either mark your answers immediately on the answer sheet, or you can mark them in the question book first of all, transferring them to the answer sheets at the end. However, if you adopt the second approach (as recommended by the Royal College) you must take great care not to run out of time, since you will not be allowed extra time to transfer marks to the answer sheet from the question book. The answer sheet must always be marked neatly and carefully according to the instructions given. Careless marking is probably one of the commonest causes of rejection of answer sheets by the document reader. For although the computer operator will do his best to interpret correctly the answer you intended and will then correct the sheet accordingly, the procedure introduces a possible new source of error. You are, of course, at liberty to change your mind by erasing your original selection and selecting a new one. In this event, your erasure should be carefully, neatly and completely carried out.

Try to leave time to go over your answers again before the end, in particular going back over any difficult questions that you wish to think about in more detail. At the same time, you can check that you have marked the answer sheet correctly. However, repeated review of your answers may in the end be counter-productive, since answers that you were originally confident were absolutely correct, often look rather less convincing at a second, third or fourth perusal. In this situation, first thoughts are usually best and too critical a revision might lead you into a state of confusion.

To guess or not to guess

Do not mark at random. Candidates are frequently uncertain whether or not to guess the answer. However, a clear distinction must be made between a genuine guess (i.e. tails for True, heads for False) and a process of reasoning by which you attempt to work out an answer that is not immediately apparent by using first principles and drawing on your knowledge and experience. Genuine guesses should not be made. You might be lucky, but if you are totally ignorant of the answer, there is an equal chance that you will be wrong and thus lose marks. This is not a chance that is worth taking and you should not hesitate to indicate 'Don't know' if this genuinely and honestly expresses your view.

Although you should not guess, you should not give in too easily. What you are doing is to increase as much as possible, the odds that the answer you are going to give is the correct one, even though you are not 100% certain that this is the case. Take time to think, therefore, drawing on first principles and reasoning power and delving into your memory stores. Do not, however, spend an inordinate amount of time on a single item that is puzzling you. Leave it, and if you have time, return to it. If you are 'fairly certain' that you know the right answer or have been able to work it out, it is reasonable to mark the answer sheet accordingly. There is a difference between being 'fairly certain' (odds better than 50:50 that you are right) and totally ignorant (where any response would be a guess). The phrase 'MCQ technique' is often mentioned and is usually used to refer specifically to this question of 'guessing' and 'Don't know'. Careful thought and reasoning ability, as well as honesty are all involved in so-called 'technique' but the best way to increase the odds that you know the right answers to the questions, is to have a sound basic knowledge of medicine and its specialties.

Trust the examiners

Do try to trust the examiners. Accept each question at its face value and do not look for hidden meanings, catches and ambiguities. Multiple Choice Questions are not designed to trick or confuse you, they are designed to test your knowledge of medicine. Don't look for problems that aren't there – the obvious meaning of a statement is the correct one and the one that you should read.

Candidates often try to calculate their score as they go through the paper; their theory is that if they reach a certain score they should then be safe in indicating 'Don't know' for any items that they have left blank without needing to take the trouble to think out answers. This approach is not to be recommended. No candidate can be certain what score he will need to achieve to obtain a pass in the examination and everyone will over-estimate the score he thinks he has obtained by answering questions confidently. The best approach is to answer every question honestly and to make every possible effort to work out the answers to more difficult questions, leaving the 'Don't know' option to indicate exactly what it means. In other words, your aim should always be to obtain the highest possible score on the MCQ paper.

The marking system

In the MCQ paper each item correctly answered is awarded one mark. For each incorrect answer one mark will be deducted. No mark is awarded or deducted for items marked 'Don't know'.

To repeat the four most important points of technique:

(1) Read the question carefully and be sure you understand it.
(2) Mark your responses clearly, correctly and accurately.
(3) Use reasoning to work out answers, but if you do not know the answer and cannot work it out, indicate 'Don't know'.
(4) The best way to obtain a good mark is to have as wide a knowledge as possible of the topics being tested in the examination.

MCQ INSTRUCTIONS

In order to help DRCOG candidates revise for the MCQ Paper we have compiled 40 questions to be used as practice material; they should not, however, be regarded as examples of actual examination questions. Each question has an answer and teaching explanation which should provide a good basis for successful revision.

We suggest that you work on this selection of 40 questions as though it were a real examination. In other words time yourself to spend no more than 1¼ hours on the practice exam and do not obtain help from books, notes or persons while working on each test. Plan to take this practice exam at a time when you will be undisturbed for a minimum of 1¼ hours. Choose a well lit location free from distractions, keep your desk clear of other books or papers, have a clock or watch clearly visible.

As you work through each question in this book be sure to mark a tick or cross (True or False) against each answer option. If you do not know the answer then leave the answer space blank.

Thus when you have completed the paper you can mark your own answers with the help of the answers and explanations given at the end of the exam. Do not be tempted to look at the questions before sitting down to take the test as this will not then represent a mock exam.

An illustration of the Opscan sheet, designed to be computer marked is shown on page 12. Reproduced with kind permission of the Royal College of Obstetricians and Gynaecologists.

Royal College of Obstetricians and Gynaecologists
Diploma Examination (DRCOG)

SURNAME

JOHNSON

INITIALS

R A

Please use HB pencil. Rub out all errors thoroughly. Mark lozenges like ▬ NOT like this ⌀ ⌀ ✗

T = True
F = False
DK = Don't know

CANDIDATE NUMBER

1	5	3	9
0	0	0	0
1 ▬	1	1	1
2	2	2	2
3	3	3 ▬	3
4	4	4	4
5	5 ▬	5	5
6	6	6	6
7	7	7	7
8	8	8	8
9	9	9	9 ▬

IMPORTANT NOTES:

1. When you have finished, check that you have NOT left any blanks and mark the DK ▬ lozenges where you Do Not Know the answer.

2. Erasures should be left clean, with no smudges where possible. (The computerised document reading machine will accept the darkest response for each item).

	A	B	C	D	E			A	B	C	D	E
1	T / F / DK	T / F / DK	T / F / DK	T / F / DK	T / F / DK		**11**	T / F / DK	T / F / DK	T / F / DK	T / F / DK	T / F / DK
2	T / F / DK	T / F / DK	T / F / DK	T / F / DK	T / F / DK		**12**	T / F / DK	T / F / DK	T / F / DK	T / F / DK	T / F / DK
3	T / F / DK	T / F / DK	T / F / DK	T / F / DK	T / F / DK		**13**	T / F / DK	T / F / DK	T / F / DK	T / F / DK	T / F / DK
4	T / F / DK	T / F / DK	T / F / DK	T / F / DK	T / F / DK		**14**	T / F / DK	T / F / DK	T / F / DK	T / F / DK	T / F / DK
5	T / F / DK	T / F / DK	T / F / DK	T / F / DK	T / F / DK		**15**	T / F / DK	T / F / DK	T / F / DK	T / F / DK	T / F / DK
6	T / F / DK	T / F / DK	T / F / DK	T / F / DK	T / F / DK		**16**	T / F / DK	T / F / DK	T / F / DK	T / F / DK	T / F / DK
7	T / F / DK	T / F / DK	T / F / DK	T / F / DK	T / F / DK		**17**	T / F / DK	T / F / DK	T / F / DK	T / F / DK	T / F / DK
8	T / F / DK	T / F / DK	T / F / DK	T / F / DK	T / F / DK		**18**	T / F / DK	T / F / DK	T / F / DK	T / F / DK	T / F / DK
9	T / F / DK	T / F / DK	T / F / DK	T / F / DK	T / F / DK		**19**	T / F / DK	T / F / DK	T / F / DK	T / F / DK	T / F / DK
10	T / F / DK	T / F / DK	T / F / DK	T / F / DK	T / F / DK		**20**	T / F / DK	T / F / DK	T / F / DK	T / F / DK	T / F / DK

A PRACTICE EXAM

40 Questions: time allowed one and a quarter hours. Indicate your answers clearly by putting a tick or cross against each answer option, or indicate 'don't know' by leaving it blank.

1. **The fetal head**

- A may be at the ischial spines but not engaged
- B can be delivered vaginally in a mento posterior position
- C will display Spalding's sign within 24 hours of intra uterine death
- D may undergo asynclitism in negotiating the pelvic outlet
- E is likely to be a vertex presentation when deflexed

2. **Regarding endometrial carcinoma**

- A endometrial carcinoma spreads to lymphatics less readily than cervical
- B radiotherapy is the treatment of choice for a pyometra (malignant)
- C in a Wertheim's hysterectomy the lower third of the vagina is excised
- D the ovaries may be conserved in the treatment of carcinoma of the corpus uteri
- E renal failure is a common cause of death in cervical carcinoma

3. **In breech presentation**

- A the perinatal morbidity is greater in the extended type
- B meconium is a reliable indicator of fetal distress
- C variable decelerations of fetal heart rate are a likely finding during intrapartum-monitoring
- D breech extraction is the method of choice for a safe vaginal delivery
- E the obstetric forceps are not necessary in multiparous patients

4. **The following conditions are thought to be commonly caused by viruses:**

A condylomata acuminata
B bartholinitis
C cervical intra-epithelial neoplasia
D lichen sclerosus
E acute vulval ulcers

5. **The following statements are true regarding cervical smears:**

A a negative result excludes frank carcinoma
B persistent inflammatory results warrant colposcopic examination
C koilocytosis is suggestive of human papilloma virus
D dyskaryosis is caused by *Trichomonas vaginalis*
E are best performed postnatally at 6 weeks

6. **A raised serum alpha-fetoprotein is likely in the following conditions:**

A spina bifida occulta
B Down's syndrome
C threatened abortion
D exomphalos
E multiple pregnancy

7. **Polyhydramnios may be associated with**

A abruptio placentae
B intra-uterine growth retardation
C fetal oesophageal atresia
D preterm labour
E postpartum haemorrhage

8. **The vaginal contraceptive diaphragm**

A is graded in 15 mm sizes
B should be removed within 2 hours of intercourse
C is recommended in cases of prolapse
D should be checked if the patient's weight changes by more than 7 lbs
E a yearly replacement is recommended

9. Endometrial carcinoma

- [ ] A is more common in obese patients
- [ ] B is a squamous carcinoma in the majority of cases
- [ ] C is more common in diabetic patients
- [ ] D can be excluded if a cervical smear is normal
- [ ] E is more common in postmenopausal women receiving cyclical oestrogen and progesterone hormone replacement therapy

10. Puerperal psychosis

- [ ] A usually begins after the second week of the puerperium
- [ ] B often takes the form of schizophrenia
- [ ] C recurrence of puerperal psychosis in subsequent pregnancies is the rule
- [ ] D the onset is usually insidious
- [ ] E the prognosis is usually good

11. Antepartum haemorrhage

- [ ] A may be secondary to a cervical erosion
- [ ] B may be treated with rest at home if the cervix is closed
- [ ] C rhesus negative patients should be given Anti-D immunoglobulin
- [ ] D there is an increased incidence of postpartum haemorrhage
- [ ] E if secondary to placental abruption, blood loss is a good indicator of severity

12. Carcinoma of the cervix

- [ ] A is the commonest malignant cause of female deaths
- [ ] B the death rate has been significantly reduced by the British screening programme
- [ ] C the majority of women dying from the condition have never had a smear
- [ ] D has a decreased incidence in smokers
- [ ] E treatment of choice is radiotherapy

13. If a pregnant woman comes into contact with rubella

- A   the majority of women will have an abnormal fetus
- B   a blood test taken immediately showing IgG antibodies means the fetus will not be affected
- C   the baby may have high tone deafness
- D   gammaglobulin should be given as soon as possible
- E   the highest risk of foetal damage occurs at 4 weeks gestation

14. The following renal changes are typical of normal pregnancy:

- A   increased glomerular filtration rate
- B   decreased excretion of urate
- C   increased excretion of folate
- D   increased excretion of glucose
- E   ureteric dilatation

15. During pregnancy

- A   glycosuria is an effective test of carbohydrate intolerance
- B   fasting plasma glucose concentration is decreased
- C   fasting plasma insulin concentration is decreased
- D   glucose tolerance alters with advancing gestation
- E   two hours after an oral glucose load, plasma insulin concentration should have returned to fasting levels

16. The volume of amniotic fluid

- A   is independent of fetal urine production
- B   may be predicted accurately by ultrasound
- C   is excessive in severe rhesus disease
- D   increases following amniocentesis
- E   is reduced in severe pre-eclampsia

17. The following factors positively influence high birth weight:

- A   maternal growth hormone
- B   prolonged pregnancy (>294 days)
- C   fetal hyperinsulinaemia
- D   primiparity
- E   social class

18. In the healthy neonate

- ☐ A the onset of physiological jaundice is between the 6th and 8th day
- ☐ B the bowel is sterile at birth
- ☐ C urine is not normally passed until 24 hours after birth
- ☐ D the respiratory rate is in the region of 25–35 per minute
- ☐ E the ductus arteriosus closes functionally within an hour of birth

19. In the fetus

- ☐ A the umbilical arteries carry oxygenated blood
- ☐ B the ductus venosus short circuits the capillaries of the liver
- ☐ C the right atrium contains a mixture of oxygenated and venous blood
- ☐ D the foramen ovale connects the ventricles of the heart
- ☐ E the ductus arteriosus joins the aorta proximal to the aortic arch

20. Pregnancy is associated with

- ☐ A an increase in cardiac output
- ☐ B a decrease in central venous pressure
- ☐ C an increase in peripheral resistance
- ☐ D an increase in pulse rate
- ☐ E a decrease in stroke volume

21. Neonatal hypocalcaemia

- ☐ A may be due to maternal dietary deficiency
- ☐ B often accompanies hypoglycaemia
- ☐ C causes permanent brain damage
- ☐ D is a common cause of convulsions
- ☐ E is seen in association with a normal maternal blood calcium concentration

22. The following drugs cross the placental barrier:

- ☐ A heparin
- ☐ B tetracycline
- ☐ C sulphadimidine
- ☐ D diazepam
- ☐ E salicylate

23. In Down's syndrome

- [ ] A most patients have an extra number 21 chromosome
- [ ] B trisomy is usually due to non-disjunction during meiosis
- [ ] C a female with Down's syndrome would never have a normal child
- [ ] D women over the age of 40 years have a risk of 1 in 200 of having a child with Down's syndrome
- [ ] E an affected fetus may be associated with a reduced serum alpha-fetoprotein concentration in amniotic fluid

24. There is a recognisable chromosome abnormality in the following:

- [ ] A Klinefelter's syndrome
- [ ] B Tay-Sachs disease
- [ ] C achondroplasia
- [ ] D Cri du chat syndrome
- [ ] E Patau's syndrome

25. Primary cytomegalovirus infection in pregnancy may cause the following in the fetus:

- [ ] A microcephaly
- [ ] B blood dyscrasias
- [ ] C myocarditis
- [ ] D pneumonia
- [ ] E enterocolitis

26. Ovulation occurs

- [ ] A before the rise in basal temperature
- [ ] B before the LH (luteinising hormone) surge
- [ ] C following follicular ripening by FSH (follicle stimulating hormone)
- [ ] D infrequently in women with amenorrhoea
- [ ] E after the disappearance of cervical mucus ferning

27. **Fetal pulmonary maturity**

   A   is delayed in diabetic pregnancies
   B   normally occurs before the 36th week of gestation
   C   is influenced by corticosteroid levels
   D   is controlled by alpha-fetoprotein
   E   is always delayed in cases of growth retardation

28. **Human chorionic gonadotrophin**

   A   is produced by the trophoblast
   B   is produced by fetal liver
   C   may be immunosuppressive
   D   reaches a peak in the second trimester of pregnancy
   E   is produced by some non-trophoblastic tumours

29. **The typical female bony pelvis**

   A   has a transverse diameter at the inlet greater than the antero-posterior diameter
   B   has an obstetric conjugate of 11–12 cm
   C   is funnel-shaped
   D   has an obtuse greater sciatic notch
   E   has a subpubic angle greater than 90°

30. **The following tumours arise in the ovary:**

   A   nephroblastoma
   B   cystadenoma
   C   granulosa cell tumour
   D   neuroblastoma
   E   teratoma

31. **In the days following ovulation**

   A   the basal body temperature falls
   B   the endometrium undergoes secretory changes
   C   the plasma progesterone concentration falls
   D   cervical mucus becomes scanty and more viscous
   E   plasma luteinising hormone level falls

32. The following genetic conditions are sex-linked:

- [ ] A the 'hairy pinna' trait
- [ ] B cleft palate
- [ ] C Hurler's syndrome (type I mucopolysaccharidosis)
- [ ] D achondroplasia
- [ ] E congenital ichthyosis

33. Common causes of meningitis in the new born include

- [ ] A *N. meningitidis*
- [ ] B *H. influenzae*
- [ ] C *E. coli*
- [ ] D group B streptococci
- [ ] E pneumococci

34. Genital herpes

- [ ] A is usually caused by the same organism as lip herpes
- [ ] B is often recurrent
- [ ] C is usually transmitted sexually
- [ ] D if uncomplicated will heal without treatment in about 10 days
- [ ] E should be treated with penicillin if secondary infection develops

35. The following micro-organisms are capable of penetrating the placenta barrier and infecting the fetus:

- [ ] A *Staphylococcus aureus*
- [ ] B *Toxoplasma gondii*
- [ ] C cytomegalovirus
- [ ] D varicella-zoster virus
- [ ] E hepatitis B virus

36. Respiratory distress syndrome of the newborn

A is always obvious at birth when present
B causes pathognomonic changes in the chest X-ray
C is unusual in full-term babies
D responds dramatically to supplementation of lung surfactants
E should be treated routinely with antibiotics

37. The use of progestogen-only contraceptives is governed by the following considerations:

A ovulation is not regularly inhibited
B protection against pregnancy is as good as with the combined pill
C there is a substantial risk in older women of venous thrombosis and embolism
D uterine bleeding may become irregular
E the dose of progestogen is much larger than in the combined pill

38. Maternal mortality is significantly increased in the presence of

A Marfan's syndrome
B valvular heart disease treated by curative surgery
C inoperable cyanotic congenital heart disease
D primary pulmonary hypertension
E congestive cardiomyopathy

39. The baby of a diabetic mother runs

A an increased risk of congenital heart disease
B a fivefold increase in risk of respiratory distress syndrome
C a 10% risk of developing diabetes
D a greatly increased risk of mental retardation
E a risk of hypomagnesaemia in the neonatal period

40. Risk factors predisposing towards maternally transmitted neonatal infection include

A prematurity
B female sex
C multiple pregnancy
D oligohydramnios
E previous reproductive loss

ANSWERS AND EXPLANATIONS TO MCQ PRACTICE EXAM

The correct answer options are given against each question.

1. **A**

   The head may be at the ischial spines when there is large caput. It is important to perform abdominal palpation at the same time as vaginal examination. A mento posterior face presentation will not be able to traverse the birth canal because flexion will not occur. Conversely in a mento anterior position flexion may result in a subsequent vaginal delivery. Spalding's sign, overlapping of the skull bones due to fetal death in utero tends to appear by about 3–7 days. Asynclitism is the phenomenom by which the head negotiates the pelvic inlet by a 'rocking' method where one parietal bone leads the other (see Chapter 6, Useful Definitions). When the head is deflexed, it is not likely to be a vertex, but a malpresentation e.g. face or brow.

2. **A E**

   Endometrial carcinoma tends to spread to lymphatics in the later stages or when there is extensive myometrial invasion. Radiotherapy is contraindicated in the presence of sepsis. Wertheim's hysterectomy entails the excision of uterus, tubes, often ovaries, upper third vagina, parametria and pelvic lymph nodes. The ovaries are excised in cases of carcinoma of the endometrium, as they are a site for malignant spread and the disease usually occurs in the postmenopausal age group. Renal failure usually occurs in carcinoma of the cervix due to the tumour obstructing both ureters.

3. **C**

   The dangers of hypoxia and fetal trauma are greater in the flexed/footling types. Meconium often reflects pressure on the fetal abdomen and is not a reliable sign of distress. Variable fetal heart rate decelerations are common due to cord compression. The technique of choice is assisted breech delivery. The obstetric forceps enable a safe delivery of the after coming head; by ensuring the head is not delivered too slowly, resulting in cerebral hypoxia, or not too rapidly, which may cause intra cranial haemorrhage (see Chapter 6 Useful Definitions).

4. **A C E**

   Condylomata acuminata are otherwise known as genital warts due to papilloma virus. Bartholinitis is usually caused by coliform organisms or staphylococci. Cervical intra-epithelial neoplasia (CIN) is thought to be caused by HPV (human papilloma virus), type 16. Lichen sclerosus is a type of vulval dystrophy of unknown aetiology. Acute vulval ulcers are most commonly due to infection by the herpes virus.

5. **B C**
A cervical smear may be negative in the presence of frank carcinoma. The surface of the malignant tissue is often ulcerated and the sample from the smear shows necrotic debris and possible inflammatory cells. A diagnosis of carcinoma can only be substantiated by cervical biopsy. Inflammatory smears do require further investigation to exclude CIN and HPV infection. Some studies have shown that 10% of inflammatory smears have CIN and >20% are associated with HPV. *Trichomonas vaginalis* may produce an inflammatory picture, which the inexperienced cytologist may find difficult to interpret, but the cells will not be dyskaryotic. Dyskaryotic cells show abnormal nuclear changes; large nuclei with increased chromatin and evidence of mitoses. Koilocytes are cells which appear 'empty' due to the presence of HPV virus within them. Cervical smears taken at the post-natal clinic at 6 weeks are notoriously inaccurate and are often obscured by inflammatory material from the lochia and necrotic tissue.

6. **C D E**
Open neural tissue in the fetus will result in passage of fetal proteins into the maternal circulation. Spina bifida occulta is a closed lesion, so this will not cause a rise in the alpha fetoprotein level. Down's syndrome may be associated with low serum levels of alpha fetoprotein. Threatened abortion may result in fetal-maternal transfusion, hence the presence of fetal blood will raise maternal serum alpha fetoprotein. Exomphalos will cause leakage of fetoprotein into amniotic fluid and by diffusion into maternal serum. Multiple pregnancy will cause a rise in alpha fetoprotein, the exact mechanism of this is unknown but presumably reflects twice as much fetal tissue.

7. **A C D E**
Abruption is a known complication of polyhydramnios which tends to occur especially when there is sudden decompression of the uterus at rupture of the membranes. It is therefore essential when performing amniotomy, to ensure that there is a slow release of the amniotic fluid. Intra-uterine growth retardation results from poor uterine blood flow which causes placental insufficiency and oligo-

hydramnios. Oesophageal atresia prevents effective fetal swallow-
ing and therefore excessive amniotic fluid forms. The over
distended uterus is more irritable and therefore prone to preterm
labour. The overstretched uterus does not retract and therefore
post-partum haemorrhage is a complication in cases of polyhydramnios.

8. D E

The diaphragm is graded in 5 mm sizes and it should be left in
position for at least 6 hours after intercourse. In cases of prolapse a
good diaphragm fitting is not possible.

9. A C

It is an adenocarcinoma, and unfortunately a negative cervical
smear does not exclude it, but it may pick up abnormal endometrial
cells. It is related to unopposed oestrogen stimulation.

10. E

Puerperal psychosis usually begins within the first 7–10 days of the
puerperium and most often takes the form of depression. Schizophrenia or mania are rare. The onset is often acute and the eventual
outcome good. The risk of recurrence in subsequent pregnancies is
between 1:3 and 1:7.

11. A C D

In antepartum haemorrhage, the patient requires hospital assessment and vaginal examination should not be performed until the
placental site is known. In placental abruption, vaginal blood loss is
not an accurate indication of severity.

12. C E

The commonest malignancy causing female deaths is breast cancer.
There has not been a significant reduction in total mortality in
Britain. The incidence of the disease is increased in smokers.

13. B C E

The highest incidence of damage is 50% at 4 weeks. The risk
decreases after the first trimester. Gammaglobulin offers no
protection from damage to the fetus and is of no value.

14. A C D E

There is an increase in the glomerular filtration rate in normal
pregnancy. This leads to an increased excretion of folate and
glucose. Because of the latter the renal threshold may be reached

and glycosuria may appear in pregnancy. Urate excretion increases by 40%. Ureteric dilatation is known to occur, possibly due to a progesterone effect.

15. B D
During pregnancy, fasting plasma glucose concentration is decreased, probably due to the haemodilution effect of the increased plasma volume. The glomerular filtration rate is increased in normal pregnancy; this may lead to the renal threshold being exceeded and to glycosuria without impaired glucose tolerance. Fasting plasma insulin concentration rises in late pregnancy to accompany the increased glucose requirements. Glucose tolerance alters during pregnancy; although plasma glucose levels should have returned to normal two hours after an oral glucose load, insulin concentration frequently remains elevated.

16. C E
From midpregnancy onwards the fetal kidney increasingly contributes to amniotic fluid volume, contributing some 500 ml per day by term; in renal agenesis the liquor volume is greatly reduced. The volume of amniotic fluid may be estimated by ultrasound, but not accurately. Liquor volumes are higher than average in rhesus affected pregnancies and grossly increased in hydrops fetalis. Amniocentesis may permit amniotic fluid to leak away, thus reducing the volume; it is not likely to increase it. Pre-eclampsia and intrauterine growth retardation are both associated with reduced amniotic fluid volumes.

17. C
There is no evidence that maternal growth hormone positively influences birth weight. Primiparity and social class are not consistently related to birth weight.

18. B D E
Physiological jaundice in a healthy baby appears after the first 48 hours of life, reaches a peak by about the fourth day and disappears within 7–10 days. The bowel is usually sterile at birth but is rapidly colonised by organisms including those encountered along the birth canal and perineum. Urine is seen to be passed in utero on ultrasound and is frequently passed at or soon after birth. The respiratory rate is usually less than 60 per minute at rest, 25–35 being usual. Constriction of the ductus arteriosus is brought about by the direct effect on the vessel wall of raising the arteriolar pO_2

with ventilation of the lungs at birth. There is probably a rapid partial closure soon after birth followed by a more gradual closure during the course of several days.

19. B C
Oxygenated blood returns from the placenta via the umbilical vein; the umbilical arteries carry deoxygenated blood from fetus to placenta. The ductus venosus provides a direct route of flow for oxygenated blood from the umbilical vein to the inferior vena cava. The foramen ovale connects the atria and is an oblique passage through the interatrial septum, which closes soon after birth due to the greater left atrial pressure closing the septum primum against the septum secundum. The ductus arteriosus is a wide channel linking the left pulmonary artery with the aorta and joins the aorta distal to the origin of the three branches of the aortic arch.

20. A D
Our understanding of the changes in cardiac output in pregnancy have evolved gradually with changes in measurement techniques. The most widely accepted view is that in the normal pregnant woman at rest, not lying supine, cardiac output rises from early pregnancy to a peak at around 20 weeks gestation which is approximately 1.5 litres per minute or 40% above the non-pregnant level; this level seems to be maintained throughout the rest of pregnancy. Although venous pressure in the legs has been shown to increase during pregnancy, that in the arms is unaltered and central venous pressure is said to remain in the range 2–5 cm water. Peripheral resistance is calculated from the mean arterial pressure divided by cardiac output; since cardiac output is increased and arterial blood pressure if anything falls slightly, it follows that peripheral resistance must be decreased. The fall has been estimated at between 20 and 40% and seems to be maximal in midpregnancy; this is due to the opening up of new vascular beds within the uterus and placenta and a general relaxation in peripheral vascular tone. The increased cardiac output of pregnancy is achieved by both an increase in heart rate (averaging 15 beats/min) and stroke volume (from 65 to 70 ml); again these changes are present from early pregnancy.

21. B D E
Calcium is actively transported across the placenta to the fetus against a concentration gradient. Soon after birth the serum calcium concentration in the baby falls, maximally on the second day. Thereafter the level rises towards adult values during the next 2–3

days. It is therefore largely unrelated to maternal blood calcium at or around birth and is unlikely to be influenced by maternal dietary deficiency. Hypocalcaemia is seen in babies born to diabetic mothers and in association with neonatal hypoglycaemia. It does not usually cause permanent brain damage, but is a common cause of neonatal tetany and/or convulsions.

22. **B C D E**
The injectable anticoagulant heparin is a large molecule and does not cross the placenta as most oral anticoagulants do and is therefore the anticoagulant of choice in pregnancy. Tetracycline is contraindicated in pregnancy because it does cross the placenta. Adverse effects include deposition in and staining of deciduous teeth and bones, tooth malformations and decrease in linear bone growth. Sulphadimidine rapidly crosses from mother to fetus. If given immediately prior to delivery there is a theoretical risk of competition between sulphonamides and bilirubin for binding sites on neonatal albumin. Diazepam readily crosses the placenta whichever route of administration is used and can cause behavioural problems for many hours after birth if given in late pregnancy or labour. Salicylates cross the placenta and can cause neonatal platelet dysfunction, decreased neonatal factor XII, neonatal haemorrhage and respiratory distress syndrome.

23. **A B E**
Down's syndrome involves an excess of chromosome 21 material but in 4% of cases this does not amount to a separate chromosome. It most frequently arises due to non-separation of the chromosomes during meiosis. A female with Down's syndrome has a 1 in 2 chance of having a normal child. After the age of 40 the risk of an affected child is more than 1 in 100. Although the diagnosis of Down's syndrome should rest upon cytological culture from placenta or amniotic fluid and genetic studies, it may be associated with reduced serum alpha fetoprotein.

24. **A D E**
Klinefelter's syndrome characteristically has an XXY chromosome complement. Cri du chat syndrome is apparently due to deletion of part of the short arm of chromosome 5. Patau's syndrome displays trisomy 13. Tay-Sachs disease is associated with a single autosomal recessive gene and achondroplasia is due to an autosomal dominant gene neither of which is normally recognisable without special techniques.

25. A B D

Primary cytomegalovirus infection during pregnancy may affect both the placenta and the fetus in up to 50% of cases. The prognosis of the infection in the fetus is not accurately known, but it is thought that such infection may produce microcephaly, choroidoretinitis, eighth nerve damage, pneumonia, hepatosplenomegaly, anaemia (sometimes haemolytic with jaundice) and intrauterine growth retardation. Myocarditis and enterocolitis are not usually associated with CMV infection.

26. A C D

Ovarian activity in humans is cyclical, the production and release of oocytes by the ovary being episodic and coordinated with its endocrine activity. FSH is largely responsible for the growth of antral follicles to maturity. The LH surge causes changes in the follicle cells of the most advanced oocyte that result in the expulsion of the oocyte at ovulation. The period prior to ovulation is characterised by oestrogen dominance, after ovulation by progestogen and oestrogen together. Both the rise in basal body temperature and the disappearance of cervical mucus ferning are attributed to the progesterone produced by the corpus luteum which forms after oocyte expulsion. Anovulation is one cause of amenorrhoea but the relationship is not absolute. Conversely regular menstruation does not necessarily indicate regular ovulation.

27. A B C

Fetal lung alveoli are lined by a group of phospholipids known collectively as 'surfactant', which prevent collapse of the alveoli during respiration by reducing surface tension. The predominant phospholipid is phosphatidyl choline (lecithin) and a surge in its production occurs at around 35 weeks gestation in normal pregnancy, promoted by glucocorticoids. Fetal lung maturity seems to be accelerated in some cases of pre-eclampsia, growth retardation and premature rupture of the membranes and is delayed in diabetes mellitus. Alpha-fetoprotein is of no relevance to pulmonary maturity.

28. A C E

Human chorionic gonadotrophin (HCG) is produced by the placental trophoblast and some other tissues but not by fetal liver. The level in maternal serum rises rapidly in early pregnancy reaching a peak between 8 and 10 weeks of pregnancy. There is then a rapid reduction to 18 weeks after which levels remain more or less constant until delivery. HCG almost certainly rescues the corpus luteum from dissolution and promotes placental steroidogenesis. It is also important in the induction of fetal testosterone secretion by Leydig cells in the male fetus. It is suggested that HCG mediates the immunological privilege afforded to the fetus. A variety of gonadal and non-gonadal tumours have been reported to produce HCG; these include tumours of the lung, stomach, liver, breast, kidney, pancreas, ovary and testis, carcinoid tumours and lymphomas.

29. A B D E
The typical female pelvic shape in the UK has a brim which is slightly wider in its transverse than A-P diameter (gynaecoid), the true obstetric conjugate being 11–12 cm and the transverse 13 cm. The cavity has the contours of a curved cylinder rather than a funnel, the side walls being approximately parallel. The greater sciatic notch is usually greater than 90° and the subpubic angle should also approximate to a right angle.

30. B C E
The cystadenoma, granulosa cell tumour and teratoma may all occur in the ovary, being derived from neoplastic growth in epithelial, sex cord and germ cell structures respectively.

The nephroblastoma and neuroblastoma are developmental tumours of kidney and nerve tissue respectively, occurring almost exclusively in early childhood and generally showing a sarcomatous appearance.

31. B D E
Basal body temperature often drops by 0.1 to 0.2°C transiently around the time of ovulation followed by a sustained rise of 0.5 to 1°C which is maintained throughout the luteal phase. The plasma LH surges to a peak around 12 hours prior to ovulation and falls progressively during the luteal phase. Plasma progesterone secretion by the corpus luteum increases to a peak around 7–8 days after ovulation and as a result the endometrium undergoes a secretory change and cervical mucus becomes more scanty, viscid and cellular.

32. A E
The term sex-linkage is virtually synonymous with X-linkage; the Y chromosome appears to have few loci apart from those determining the male sex. The only documented Y-linked state is that of the 'hairy pinna'.

Congenital ichthyosis is an X-linked disorder associated with a steroid sulphatase deficiency (and hence may be associated with very low oestriol levels in pregnancy).

Hurler's syndrome is determined by an autosomal recessive gene and achondroplasia by an autosomal dominant. Cleft palate, whether or not associated with cleft lip, seems to have a multi-factorial inheritance pattern.

33. C D
The organisms commonly responsible for meningitis in children and adults are relatively uncommon as a cause among the newborn.

34. B C D
Genital herpes is usually caused by *Herpes virus hominis* Type II whereas ordinary lip herpes is caused by *H. hominis* Type I. Penicillin and other treponemicidal drugs should NOT be given as they may confuse the diagnosis of coincidental syphilis.

35. B C D E
The placental barrier is completely effective against nearly all bacterial and protozoal invaders (*Toxoplasma* is an exception) and in general only viruses can cross it.

36. C
The baby may appear well immediately after birth; signs usually develop within 1–2 hours. The chest X-ray appearances are suggestive but not pathognomonic. Treatment with surfactants has no effect and antibiotics are not indicated.

37. A D
The progestogen-only pill is less effective than the combined pill but there are no serious adverse effects. The dose of progestogen is much smaller than the combined pill.

38. A C D E
Patients who have undergone curative cardiac surgery are at no increased risk. The remaining conditions are all associated with increased maternal mortality and are grounds for avoiding pregnancy altogether.

39. A B E
The risk of the child developing diabetes is thought to be between 1% and 5%. Mental retardation is uncommon. The blood levels of

both calcium and magnesium may fall significantly during the first 3 days of life if the mother is being treated with insulin; this is thought to be due to delayed development of the baby's parathyroid function.

40. A C E
Male sex and polyhydramnios are risk factors.

THE ESSAY QUESTION PAPER

It is quite likely that you may not have written an essay for many years and it is wise to practise before the exam. Initially pick a topic to which you know the answer and write a leisurely answer without reference to the time. You will be horrified at the result! When you have gained experience and confidence limit your answer to the 45 minutes allowed in the exam, then progress to practising with past papers, asking your consultant to go over them with you. It can take quite some time to become confident and fluent with your answers so start a good three months before the exam.

In the examination there are two compulsory essay questions to be answered in one and a half hours. Each question must be answered in a separate book and answers should be written legibly on the right-hand pages only. No part of the book should be torn out. (Any work you wish to discard should have a line drawn through it.) Candidates are advised that the essay questions are not only designed to assess knowledge but the ability to develop arguments, discussion and communicate in written English. Marks are lost for poor presentation, particularly if answers are not presented as essays. It is essential that writing is legible and marks will be lost if examiners are unable to read candidates' scripts.

1. Read each question slowly and deliberately. Each question has key words to concentrate the scope of your answer; underline these words. Make sure you are quite clear what the examiner is asking for, *no marks are given for parts of answers not relevant to the question asked.* If for example a question asks how you would manage a certain condition, do not write at length about its aetiology, pathology or prevention no matter how well you know it and how well it might flow from the pen, they are asking *how you would deal with it* when it has occurred.

2. Always attempt an answer however little you may know. If you write nothing you will get no marks for that question and with the 'close' marking system in use you will fail.

3. Before deciding how to set out your answer it is useful to consider the examiner's view. The examiner is only human, despite rumours to the contrary, and he wishes to know if you have:

   a) understood the question

    b) analysed the components of the question logically

    c) assessed the relative importance and priority of these components

    d) answered the question concisely without irrelevant deviations, taking account of alternative points of view where applicable

    e) presented the answer legibly

The examiner will take into account the time limit, the stress the examination causes and that you are not as well versed in the subject as he is.

With these points in mind you can approach the answer. It is unnecessary to write out the question at the beginning of your answer, do not waste your time.

Write a skeleton plan of your answer on the left-hand pages provided for rough work. This will ensure you do not omit any important points in your definitive answer, it will also give the examiner a rapid clue as to whether you have included the relevant points.

You should be paying constant attention to the time. Allow 45 minutes for each question and do not overrun on the first question as this will jeopardize your answer to the second question which could leave you insufficient time to present an adequate answer on the last question to achieve a pass mark. Both questions carry equal marks and need their full time quota. Each question is marked by one pair of examiners, they do not know how you have performed in the other question and will make no allowance.

Answer the questions in the order in which you are most confident. Of the 45 minutes allowed for each question you should spend the first 5 minutes making sure you have understood the question and identifying the key words, then a further 10–15 minutes working on the skeleton, leaving 25–30 minutes to write down the definitive answer. This should be about 600–700 words long.

If you do not think you know much about a particular question do not despair. Leave it to last and approach the individual components of the question from first principles. Most questions are very practical in their orientation so think back to how you dealt with that situation when you were doing your SHO job, or how you would deal with it in the surgery. It is not possible in a book of this nature to cover all possibilities in detail, however, by tackling each of the following essay questions in turn and by comparing your efforts with the model full length essays provided you should be able to polish up your technique and improve your presentation.

Remember that the best answers are not necessarily the longest. By careful analysis of the question, consideration of the components and concise presentation you are more likely to get your points across to the examiner than by an ill considered, poorly presented jumble of ideas.

Write legibly. Illegible scrawl causes 'examiner stress' and loses marks. Keep to simple language with reasonable punctuation. It is surprising how poor the grammar is in the average answer, often a result of lack of practise and frequent use of abbreviations and 'case-note' English.

For ease of reading, the underlining of subheadings and the provision of breaks between paragraphs is preferable to an homogeneous mass of script with one point merging almost imperceptibly into the next. Avoid using the first person in your answer unless the question specifically asks for *your* management of a situation. Standard abbreviations may be used after their first use but avoid 'case note' abbreviations.

The Marking System

Each part of the examination (written, clinical and oral) is marked out of 100 with a pass mark of 51.

In the written examination 50 marks are allocated to the MCQ paper and 50 marks to the Essay Question Paper. Each essay question is marked by two examiners on a basis of 25 marks per question. The marks given are in the range 11–14.

A mark of 14 indicates an excellent answer.
A mark of 13 is a pass mark beyond doubt.
A mark of 12 indicates a fail answer (average undergraduate answer).
A mark of 11 indicates fail by any standard.

Acknowledgement

The authors are very grateful to the Royal College for their permission to use past essay questions as studied on the following pages.

SAMPLE ESSAY QUESTIONS WITH MODEL ANSWERS

In the DRCOG examination there will be two compulsory essay questions to be answered in 1½ hours.

SAMPLE ESSAY QUESTIONS: OBSTETRICS

1. How is the perinatal mortality rate defined? What are the main causes of perinatal mortality? What changes have contributed to the reduction in perinatal mortality in the last twenty years?

This is a straightforward factual question. However, you should bear in mind that there is a substantial geographical variation in causes which should be mentioned, although your answer to the last part of the question should be mainly concerned with the United Kingdom.

Key words: main causes; changes; twenty years.

Rough outline:

Definition

main causes: prematurity; malformations; infection; APH; trauma; unexplained.

changes: improved general health and living conditions, including diet; improved health education; screening for abnormality; closer monitoring in labour and earlier intervention where necessary; improved neonatal techniques.

Model answer:

The perinatal mortality rate is defined as the number of stillbirths occurring after 28 weeks gestation plus the number of deaths occurring in the first week of life divided by the total number of stillbirths plus live births, expressed as a rate per thousand total births.

The main causes of perinatal mortality vary in different parts of the world, particularly the role of infection which is small in the United Kingdom and the incidence of lethal congenital malformations which are less important because of early diagnosis allowing termination of pregnancy.

36

In the United Kingdom at present the main causes are prematurity accounting for some 25–30% of deaths despite the marked improvements in paediatric intensive care. Pregnancy complications which result in chronic or acute fetal asphyxia such as antepartum haemorrhage and pregnancy induced hypertension account for 15–25%. (If one considers countries where termination of pregnancy is not available, malformations account for up to 30% of cases.) It is significant that these leading causes are all more commonly seen in the same group, namely the lower socio-economic and high parity families.

Birth trauma accounts for 5–10% of deaths although recently it has been suggested that a number of cases claimed to be a result of birth trauma can be shown to have evidence of earlier problems. With further development of ultrasound techniques and facilities this may become clearer. Infection is a small problem accounting for only 1–2%. There remains a significant group of unexplained cases which may be as high as 20%.

The perinatal mortality rate has fallen dramatically over the past twenty years and we are now reaching the point where further improvement of even modest degree will need considerable effort. There are many factors involved in this improvement.

The prevention and successful treatment of infections brought about a big fall, not merely because of antibiotics but because of improvement in the general health and living standards of the population (although the higher proportion of deaths is still in the less privileged groups). There is better health education and pregnant women are more aware of the need for good nutrition, avoidance of cigarettes, alcohol and drugs etc.

The availability of ultrasound and serum screening tests and the introduction of the 1967 Abortion Act have reduced the incidence of fetal abnormalities, although this still represents fetal wastage as the underlying problem remains.

The ability to suppress preterm labour, the maturation of fetal lungs and establishment of neonatal intensive care facilities have reduced the problem of prematurity, or rather have allowed more babies born earlier to have a chance of survival. The outlook for a fetus of 27–28 weeks born today is probably better than that for one born at 32 weeks twenty years ago. (The long term outlook for the very immature infants, less than 26 weeks, remains uncertain, a number die later transferring the death from the perinatal group to the infant mortality figures.)

Improved monitoring of the fetus during labour with electronic and biochemical methods for high risk situations, and the ability to induce and augment labour where the fetus is at risk has led to a fall in asphyxial deaths. Recognition that there is no excuse for a 'traumatic' vaginal delivery with prompt recourse to Caesarean section either before or during labour has reduced the incidence of 'traumatic' deaths.

Despite the impressive improvements (achieved mainly in intra and postpartum deaths rather than stillbirths) there can be no room for complacency especially when one considers that still some 40% of perinatal deaths occur in infants born after 37 weeks gestation and weighing over 2500 grams.

2. Outline the methods currently available for the antenatal diagnosis of fetal abnormality. A woman of 40 presents with eight weeks amenorrhoea and a positive pregnancy test. How would you counsel her?

Key words: outline; currently available; antenatal; 40; eight weeks; you; counsel.

This is a specific question with a relatively narrow scope which tests both your knowledge of the subject and your approach to a particular situation. Note that the first part of the question asks for an outline of currently available methods. The second part asks how you would counsel her, so you must discuss your approach not an impersonal possible approach. This answer will fill the 45 minute time allocation, beware of overrunning.

Rough outline:

History:

> previous abnormality
> family history of congenital abnormality
> medical history, drugs, alcohol, infections, diabetes, age

Investigations:

> CVS
> AFP
> ultrasound
> amniocentesis (anti D)
> fetoscopy and cordocentesis

Counselling:

> ?planned pregnancy
> ?acceptance of TOP if abnormal
> risk of abnormality
> incidence of malformations
> investigations available, what they can detect and what they will not detect, inherent risk of complications, time until results available.

Model answer:

In order to make a diagnosis one would start with the history, looking in particular for:

a history of any previous abnormality
a family history of congenital abnormality, medical history and medication, alcohol intake, infections, diabetes, particularly during the first 8 weeks after conception.
age of mother

If the parents would seek a termination of the pregnancy where a major abnormality is detected the diagnosis needs to be made as soon as possible. In early pregnancy clinical examination is unlikely to give much help unless there is a history of exposure to infection or where glycosuria is found on routine testing.

The special investigations currently available to detect the common abnormalities include:

Chorionic villus sampling (CVS); a recent technique which allows chromosome studies to be performed on a small sample of chorionic tissue obtained either transabdominally or transcervically under ultrasound guidance at around 10 weeks, thus permitting a suction termination where appropriate. As yet it is not widely available and its risks are uncertain. Clinical trials are still being conducted.

Serum alpha fetoprotein (AFP) levels. AFP is produced by the developing fetus and can be measured in maternal serum. Normal ranges have been established for between 16 and 20 weeks and elevated levels indicate the need for closer assessment. It is only a screening test and is not very specific. Possible causes of a raised level include:

wrong dates
multiple pregnancy
a recent bleed
open neural tube defects
abdominal wall defects
vascular anomalies in placenta or cord

Where no abnormality is subsequently found in the presence of a persistently raised level there appears to be an increased risk of intrauterine growth retardation, the reason for which is unknown.

Very low levels have been claimed to be associated with an increased risk of Down's syndrome especially where the maternal levels of HCG and oestriol are also estimated and the results interpreted in relation to the maternal age. Further studies in this area are awaited as it may help

40

improve the pick up rate, considering that some 75% of all Down's syndrome infants are born to women in the so called low risk group.

Ultrasound. In most obstetric units an ultrasound examination is offered to all pregnant women at around 16 to 20 weeks gestation. Depending upon the facilities and expertise available this examination can yield much information about the fetus. At the least it confirms the maturity and viability of the pregnancy and excludes multiple pregnancy. It should also detect major skeletal abnormalities including anencephaly, open neural tube defects, limb problems and renal absence. As the techniques develop it is becoming possible to detect more subtle abnormalities and even 'markers' for chromosomal abnormalities. However, such examinations require sophisticated equipment, great expertise and time.

Amniocentesis. By examination of either cells or fluid components of amniotic fluid at around 16–20 weeks it is possible to detect over 100 different abnormalities. Almost all of them involve complex time consuming and expensive tests and are only applicable in a small number of cases where there is a particularly high risk of a rare condition.

The majority of amniocentesis tests are performed to look for chromosomal abnormalities or to confirm the presence of neural tube defects in the presence of raised AFP levels (however with present scan quality and operator expertise almost all open defects can be visualised and the need for amniocentesis in these cases is falling).

The risk of a chromosomal abnormality rises with maternal age and most hospitals have a policy of offering the test to all pregnant women above a predetermined age (depending upon local facilities) in most places this is 35 years and over.

The procedure involves passing a needle transabdominally into the amniotic sac under ultrasound guidance and withdrawing 10–20 ml of amniotic fluid. There is a risk of complications, miscarriage, infection or rarely fetal injury in up to 1% of cases. In all cases the woman's rhesus factor should be known and anti D immunoglobulin given to rhesus negative women to avoid the sensitisation.

Cordocentesis and fetoscopy are new developments which permit visualisation of the fetus via a small telescope permitting samples of fetal blood to be taken from the umbilical cord under ultrasound direction. The latter technique has been used to detect haemoglobinopathies.

Counselling the woman.

For this 40 year old the particular points which come to mind are that in addition to the 2–3% incidence of fetal abnormality in the general population she is at increased risk of a chromosomal abnormality in respect of her age. The risk of Down's syndrome is about 1 in 90 if there is no significant history. At eight weeks she is early enough for CVS if available.

I would ask her if it were a planned pregnancy and if so if there had been any delay in conceiving. I would discuss with her (and her partner if he cared to come) the anticipated course of pregnancy in a woman of 40 with particular reference to any relevant medical, obstetrical or family history. I would then discuss the question of increased risk of chromosomal abnormalities against the perspective of the overall incidence of abnormalities and would discuss the diagnostic tests available as described above, pointing out that the tests only exclude the conditions looked for and that there is no way to guarantee a 'perfect' baby.

I would ask if they would seek termination of the pregnancy if the fetus were found to be abnormal. If they would not consider it then there is no point in subjecting mother (and fetus) to an unnecessary risk of CVS or amniocentesis. Serum AFP levels would not be appropriate either. If they would seek termination I would discuss in detail the chances of the abnormality occurring and of the proposed test, explaining what the test involves, how long it is likely to be before the results are available and to answer any questions they have about either the possible abnormalities or the tests.

I believe that the final decision as to whether to have the tests rests with the couple when they are in possession of the relevant facts and I would not try to press my views on to them or even tell them what I would do in similar circumstances.

If they wish to go ahead I would refer them to the specialist, requesting an early appointment, particularly if CVS might be considered.

3. You are a General Practitioner in charge of patients in an isolated GP maternity unit 15 miles from the nearest consultant obstetric unit. How would you manage a patient with:

1. **Cord prolapse**

2. **Primary postpartum haemorrhage**

This is a very clear specific question defining precisely a given set of circumstances. It tests your ability to cope with emergency situations in isolation.

It is no use wasting time writing about philosophical considerations of the advisability of having such isolated units or that you would not use such a unit. Nor should you waste time on discussing prophylactic measures other than selection criteria for delivery in such a unit. For the purposes of your answer the problem has arisen, you are 15 miles away from the main unit and you must describe how you would deal with the situation.

The answer can be quite concise and you should finish comfortably within the 45 minutes if you restrict yourself to answering the question asked. Indeed you could answer the question in two or three paragraphs outlining immediate action and summoning the flying squad! However, one must recognise the practicalities of obstetrics and that it is virtually impossible for a consultant unit to be able to guarantee to respond immediately at any time to a call for the flying squad.

Key words: isolated; 15 miles

Rough outline:

> selection criteria to exclude potentially high risk women; parity, previous obstetric history.
>
> problems arising in pregnancy; polyhydramnios, large baby, unstable lie, high head.

cord prolapse
> push up to avoid compression, keep cord in vagina, speak to registrar, ?facilities in unit for LSCS, ?availability of flying squad, ?better to escort patient to main unit.

PPH:
> haemostasis, IV ergometrine, IV oxytocin

resuscitation, IV infusions, blood for cross match, volume expanders, catheter
determine cause, ?retained tissue, ?trauma, ?atonic, ?DIC, ?local theatre facilities
contact registrar, ?availability of flying squad, ?escort in

Model answer:

Cord prolapse occurs when the membranes rupture with the cervix dilating and no presenting part in the pelvis or covering the os. It is more likely to occur in multiparous women, where there is cephalopelvic disproportion, an unstable lie, or malpresentation and when the presenting part is high at term.

When booking a woman for delivery in an isolated unit one must apply strict selection criteria to minimise the risks of complications arising away from the back-up facilities of a consultant unit. Thus one would not book grand multipara or those with a history of large babies or recurrent unstable lie in a previous pregnancy. During the course of the pregnancy one would transfer the booking if abnormalities arose. Having done all one can to reduce the risk to a minimum, cord prolapse will still occasionally occur.

Upon making the diagnosis, usually at vaginal examination the important thing is to prevent compression of the cord between the presenting part and the pelvis by pushing upward on the presenting part and keeping the cord within the vagina to prevent vascular spasm in the colder environment. This is helped by tipping the bed into a head down position so that gravity assists in preventing cord compression. Use of the knee-chest position is awkward, undignified and less effective than simply tipping the bed. If the cord is not pulsating the child is already dead and arrangements can be made to transfer the mother to the main unit by local ambulance.

Assuming the cord is still pulsating the presenting part must be kept off the cord, I would ask the midwife in attendance to take over this task allowing me to contact the senior resident doctor on duty at the consultant unit.

The action taken will depend upon a number of factors.

Are there facilities at the GP unit to perform a Caesarean section?

Local policy agreed between GPs and Consultant unit staff on when the flying squad should go out and when the patient should be transferred in.

Availability of staff at the consultant unit to respond to a flying squad call. In the majority of consultant units the staff can be very busy with obstetric and gynaecological emergencies and if they are in theatre performing a caesarean section or dealing with an ectopic they will be unable to come out. In addition, where the obstetric staff are free to respond the anaesthetist may not be, as many hospitals still do not have anaesthetic registrars with sole responsibility for the maternity unit at all times. A flying squad call takes most of the experienced on-call staff away from the busy main unit and in many circumstances it may be more appropriate and quicker to transfer the mother to the consultant unit directly rather than via a flying squad call.

Post partum haemorrhage

In selecting women for delivery in the GP unit one would exclude those at increased risk of a postpartum haemorrhage, including those with a history of

retained placenta
postpartum haemorrhage
high parity.

During pregnancy the development of polyhydramnios, unstable lie, a large baby would determine a transfer of booking.

Once a primary postpartum haemorrhage has occurred prompt action is essential and the following steps occur almost simultaneously. It is essential to control the bleeding and maintain the circulation to prevent the complications of acute renal failure and anterior pituitary necrosis and death. The management depends to some extent upon the cause, thus oxytocics are of little use if the bleeding is from a vaginal or cervical tear, or in the presence of a coagulation failure. If the placenta is retained it may be possible to remove it from the cervix if it is separated. Most cases of primary haemorrhage are associate with uterine atony.

An intravenous infusion must be set up with a large bore cannula, taking blood for subsequent cross-match. An intravenous injection of 0.5 mg ergometrine should be given followed by an infusion of 100 units of oxytocin in a litre of Hartman's solution at 40 drops per minute. The circulation should be maintained with plasma volume expanders after blood has been taken for cross match. A urethral catheter should be inserted to monitor urine output.

Unless there is an IMMEDIATE response arrangements must be made to transfer the woman to the main unit (if it is a retained placenta this could be removed in the GP unit by the flying squad, tears could be sutured if adequate facilities exist on site). In some areas other GPs administer anaesthetics and theoretically this would permit more to be done on site but in the majority of cases transfer of the woman to the consultant unit with all its back up facilities readily available is best.

The question as to whether the flying squad are summoned, or their ability to respond, or whether the mother should be transferred to the hospital directly is as discussed above in relation to cord prolapse.

4. Discuss with examples, the factors which influence you when prescribing drugs during the antenatal period and in the puerperium.

At first sight a broad question but in fact the underlying considerations can be expressed concisely and a comfortable pass achieved well within the 45 minutes.

Key words: examples; you; prescribing; antenatal period; puerperium

Rough outline:

first week, abortion or no effect
up to eight weeks, physical abnormalities
later, growth or functional development effects
labour, respiratory problems, feeding problems, behavioural problems; jaundice

risk difficult to assess
impossible to guarantee safety
prescribe only if absolute need
use established drugs
lowest dose
shortest time
up to date info

Model answer:

Over the past 20 years there has been an increasing awareness and concern about the possibility of adverse effects upon the fetus from drugs given to the mother. This has been highlighted, although rather distorted, by the thalidomide and diethyl stilboestrol cases. It is very difficult to assess the risk of adverse effects from a particular drug for several reasons, including:

lack of human data
species differences in susceptibility
prevalence of abnormalities anyway at 2–3% of all deliveries
variable individual response (only 25% of fetuses exposed to thalidomide were affected)

It is currently believed that drug induced effects have very little influence on the prevalence of abnormalities.

Adverse effects in the first week after conception will either cause an abortion or damaged cells will be replaced by other undifferentiated cells and develop normally.

Thereafter, up to eight weeks, the various organs and systems are differentiating and adverse effects will cause congenital abnormalities in the systems differentiating at the time of exposure (e.g. corticosteroids may cause cleft lip or palate).

Beyond eight weeks adverse effects may affect growth or functional development (opiate addiction, smoking).

Anticoagulants are a suitable example of oral agents taken in the first eight weeks which may cause abnormalities, i.e. fetal warfarin syndrome later in pregnancy. The use of oral agents may cause fetal haemorrhage and there is a fetal loss rate of up to 15%. Heparin does not cross the placenta and is therefore safe. However, prolonged use may cause maternal osteoporosis.

Drugs taken shortly before delivery may affect neonatal respiration (opiates in labour) and feeding, or cause behavioural changes (diazepam, insulin) or cause jaundice (sodium benzoate in diazepam injections, sulphonamides, high doses of oxytocin).

For the breast-feeding woman there is more information available from human studies and it is easy to measure drug levels in milk. The pharmacokinetics of drug excretion in milk and absorption are well documented and there are readily available sources of frequently updated information for one to consult. A number of drugs are contraindicated in breast feeding, e.g. tetracyclines can affect dental and bone formation. In addition to breast feeding, the puerperium and the use of drugs can also produce problems e.g. the use of oestrogens for suppression of lactation or contraception may produce thromboembolism. Drugs may be necessary to suppress lactation, e.g. bromocryptine.

An example which demonstrates the above principles is the use of anticoagulants. Oral anticogulants, e.g. warfarin, are teratogenic if used in early pregnancy and are excreted in breast milk, with the risk of neonatal haemorrhage. Heparin, however, does not cross the placenta and is preferable in early and late pregnancy.

The only drug known to cause *maternal* problems is oestrogen if given to suppress lactation. Thromboembolic phenomena may occur. This does not occur with combined oral contraceptives but these may suppress lactation.

Although the risk of serious adverse effects appears to be small it is impossible to guarantee the safety of a particular drug and I therefore follow these guidelines:

I only prescribe when there is an absolute indication and where the beneficial effects anticipated outweigh the theoretical adverse effects.

I would use established drugs rather than recently introduced drugs where effects may not yet have been recognised.

I would prescribe the lowest effective dose for the shortest effective duration and I would consult the most up to date information available (e.g. BNF, the Boehringer Ingelheim Drugs in Breast Milk chart).

5. What might lead you to suspect a multiple pregnancy before the 20th week of gestation? Discuss how the problems that may be encountered antenatally influence your advice to and management of the patient expecting twins.

A straightforward uncomplicated question which can be answered satisfactorily well within the time. Avoid the temptation to 'fill in' with material irrelevant to the question asked.

Key words: suspect; before 20th week; antenatally

Rough outline:

> history, previous and both families
> ethnic group
> induced ovulation/GIFT/IVF
> increased symptoms
> uterine size
>
> problems: anaemia; smaller babies; PPH; preterm labour; polyhydramnios; unstable lie
>
> management: work; rest; smoking; diet; iron and folate; check presenting part/cervix

Model answer:

The presence of a multiple pregnancy may be suspected in those women who are at increased risk including those who have previously had a multiple pregnancy or where there is a family history on either side. Where ovulation has been induced, particularly with gonadotrophin therapy, or where pregnancy followed the use of in vitro fertilisation or gamete intra Fallopian transfer techniques there is an increased risk. Women from negroid races have a higher incidence of multiple pregnancy. Where there is no obvious 'risk' factor the condition may be suspected if she is experiencing an exaggeration of early pregnancy symptoms, especially nausea. A uterus which is larger than expected for the dates may be found but this is more commonly seen after 20 weeks.

Women with multiple pregnancies are prone to a number of antenatal problems which should be looked for. It is quite in order for women with twin pregnancies to have shared antenatal care between consultant unit and GP. Communication between the two will establish the desired frequency of visits to each.

Anaemia is more common, both iron deficiency and folate deficiency (as more folate is required for the increased DNA synthesis), regular full blood count estimations should be made through the pregnancy looking at the indices to detect potential deficiencies before the haemoglobin falls. In addition to oral iron supplements, folate should be given in a dose of 5 mg twice daily, rather than the 350 micrograms found in the combined preparations.

Twins tend to be smaller than singletons and the mother should be encouraged to take a balanced diet, cut out smoking where applicable, take periods of rest and finish work earlier than with a singleton. It is appropriate to perform ultrasound scans in the third trimester to detect evidence of growth retardation.

Preterm labour is more common, perhaps related to increased uterine distension, particularly if there is polyhydramnios. She should be warned of this risk and advised to plan her domestic arrangements to permit more rest, finishing work early where appropriate, not to plan distant trips, especially overseas. Although there is no need for prophylactic hospital-isation for the majority of women with twins, they must attend frequently for antenatal checks, looking especially for signs of imminent preterm labour. Early descent of the presenting part into the pelvis indicates the need to check the cervix for signs of effacement or dilatation. If there is any suspicion that preterm labour is imminent admission is indicated.

Pregnancy induced hypertension is more common particularly in first pregnancies, this should be looked for.

Unstable lie is more common owing to uterine distension and the increased placental size increases the chances of placenta praevia. Placental location by ultrasound is indicated if there is unstable lie.

It is held that the 'placental reserves' do not permit the fetuses to cope with prolonged pregnancy and if labour has not ensued it is still usual for labour to be induced at term.

6. Discuss the diagnosis and implications of sexually transmitted disease in pregnancy.

A topical question in light of recent publicity surrounding HIV infections. Rather loose in its scope it should nevertheless be possible to give a comprehensive answer within the time allowed.

Key words: diagnosis; implications; sexually transmitted; during pregnancy

Rough outline:

diagnosis: often symptom free

history of contact; high risk woman; vaginal discharge

swabs; blood tests; implications of screening

implications: risk to fetus in utero or during delivery; immediate or long term; risk to attendants

gonorrhoea (GC); herpes; syphilis; trichomonas vaginitis (TV); non-specific urethritis (NSU); AIDS; chlamydia

Model answer:

Many women suffering from an existing sexually transmitted disease, or contracting one during pregnancy are symptom free which makes diagnosis less simple. One needs to maintain an awareness of the possibility and a high index of suspicion, particularly where the woman is considered to be at increased risk.

The history taken when the woman is 'booked' should include relevant details including the history of previous terminations of pregnancy, ectopic pregnancies, pelvic inflammatory disease or sexually transmitted disease. A history of drug abuse is also important. Often the woman may wish to suppress important details and here the family practitioner has an important role as he is more likely to be aware of the overall picture. She may disclose symptoms suggestive of a current or recent infection such as vaginal discharge (although this is a common complaint in pregnancy and monilial infections are also more common) or blisters or ulcers on the labia suggesting a herpes infection.

Where the history or clinical findings raise the possibility of infection the appropriate swabs should be sent for culture.

Most hospitals perform routine serological screening tests for syphilis, the question as to their cost effectiveness today is being debated. The actual tests done vary between centres, most relying on the VDRL as a screen and performing confirmatory tests where this is positive. Serological tests for gonorrhoea have been abandoned as they are inaccurate. Routine high vaginal and cervical swabs are not commonly performed except for high risk women.

The question of screening for HIV has been widely debated and the present view is that this should only be done with the consent of the woman and not otherwise. There has yet to be public debate on the current established screening tests which it could be argued should follow the same criteria.

The implications of an untreated STD affect mainly the fetus which may be infected in utero or during delivery. Paediatricians need to be informed ready to act urgently to treat the neonate. If one considers the common diseases these risks become apparent.

Gonorrhoea might affect the fetus during delivery giving rise to ophthalmia neonatorum. Syphilis may cause stillbirth or late abortion or the child may be born with stigmata of congenital disease such as the typical facial appearance. Trichomonas does not usually cause many problems. Monilia may affect the fetus during delivery and cause infection. Herpes virus is a potentially serious problem. Ascending infection can affect the fetus once membrane rupture has occurred. Neonatal herpes is often fatal and if cultures or electron microscopy studies show the shedding of virus particles at term delivery by caesarean section is recommended before the onset of labour or before the membranes rupture. Other infections transmitted sexually can affect fetal development e.g. chlamydia, cytomegalovirus, toxoplasmosis.

Acquired immune deficiency syndrome resulting from infection with HIV has received widespread publicity. The extent of the problem is uncertain. It is a highly lethal condition and there is no cure. The virus can affect the fetus in utero. With the present policy regarding screening and the difficulty in interpreting the results where screening is performed the only practical approach is to take sensible precautions when dealing with any fluids or secretions. The risk of attendants contracting the disease is probably small but is as yet uncertain. If the numbers of confirmed cases continues to rise at the present rate it is not unreasonable to foresee a dramatic change in the approach to childbirth, having spent the last few years making the whole process more 'natural' the prospect of wearing protective clothing, goggles and masks for deliveries may well be met with much resistance by the public.

SAMPLE ESSAY QUESTIONS: GYNAECOLOGY

7. An elderly lady presents with urinary incontinence and urgency of micturition. Discuss the possible causes of these complaints and the management of such a patient.

This is a typical 'compound' question covering a broad field giving wide scope for the answer but providing a few clues as to the more likely causes. It is difficult to give a precise answer because of this lack of detail.

It is the type of question designed to see if you have a grasp of the overall topic of urinary problems in the elderly. Beware of the temptation to go into detail on one aspect at the expense of 'covering the field'. You will find that the answer takes all of the 45 minutes you should allocate, avoid the temptation to overrun the time.

Key words: elderly; urinary incontinence and urgency; possible causes; management.

Rough outline:

> difficult to obtain clear history
> mixture of symptoms

Possible causes:

> atrophic urethrotrigonitis
> detrusor instability
> habit
> genuine stress incontinence
> overflow incontinence
> loss of social awareness

Management:

> obtain history as far as possible, looking for:
> type of incontinence, stress or urge frequency, urgency, nocturia, dysuria, hesitancy or flow problems.

Clinical examination, looking for:

> general condition, physical and mental, vaginal atrophy, descent of bladder neck, stress incontinence, tenderness over urethra and trigone, MSSU.

54

Model answer:

The possible causes of urgency and incontinence include:

a) atrophic urethrotrigonitis where the epithelium of the urethra and trigone become atrophic owing to the lack of oestrogen post-menopausally. Being derived from similar embryological areas to the vagina they are similarly oestrogen sensitive

b) detrusor instability whether secondary to chronic inflammation as following oestrogen lack, especially if there is an associated urethral stenosis, or not. Bladder calculi may also present in this way

c) habit deriving from a previous inflammatory or instability problem, now resolved

d) overflow incontinence may occur with chronic retention. This may be seen secondary to urethral stenosis or may be the result of a chronic loss of awareness of the desire to micturate, leading to a large capacity, atonic bladder. Overflow into the urethra may stimulate a desire to micturate interpreted as urgency

e) genuine stress incontinence associated with a weakness of the sphincter mechanism. This would not account for the urgency, but is often part of a 'mixed' pattern of symptoms

f) a loss of social awareness found with dementia may present as incontinence, the lady being unaware of the social need to control bladder function. However, it is unlikely that she would present of her own volition or complain of urgency.

In order to decide which condition(s) one is dealing with an accurate history is necessary. However, this is not always possible with an elderly lady, especially if she is confused or suffering from dementia.

One would like to know whether the incontinence is genuine stress incontinence or urge incontinence. Also, any additional urinary symptoms should be determined, including frequency, nocturia, dysuria or haematuria which might point to an inflammatory cause or detrusor instability. Hesitancy and a history of poor flow and a sensation of incomplete emptying are often found in cases of urethral stenosis.

Details of her past obstetric history may be significant if there is a history of stress incontinence. A history of recurrent 'cystitis' may suggest an inflammatory factor or the basis of a habit problem. In the presence of dysuria the site of the pain can be helpful, suprapubic pain suggesting a bladder or trigonal origin, vaginal pain a urethral origin.

On clinical examination one should check for bladder distension, suprapubic tenderness, vaginal atrophy, prolapse of the urethral mucosa, any descent of the bladder neck and evidence of genuine stress incontinence and any tenderness on palpating the urethra and trigone. A mid stream specimen of urine should be examined to exclude infection. Any evidence of pelvic pathology should be sought.

Asking a lady who is able to cooperate to keep a frequency/volume chart can be helpful.

The management depends upon the diagnosis and its underlying cause.

One of the commonest causes of the combination of symptoms is likely to be a chronic atrophic condition. For these women any urinary infection should be treated according to bacteriological sensitivities. If there is no growth low dose antibiotic therapy such as trimethoprim 100 mg or nitrofurantoin 50 mg taken each night for two months and local oestrogen therapy (as cream or pessaries) used twice weekly on a long term basis often brings about a marked improvement. If there is no improvement in three months or if there is a suggestion of urethral stenosis which requires urethral dilatation, referral is indicated.

If one suspects stress incontinence, particularly in the presence of visible descent of the bladder neck, a ring pessary may provide relief, aided by weight reduction where appropriate. In fit women where surgery would be acceptable referral to a specialist is indicated.

If detrusor instability is suspected one could prescribe either anticholinergics or one of the newer calcium blockers such as terodilin taken orally 12.5–25 mg bd. Discussion with the local specialist is often helpful to decide upon the need for urodynamic investigations to provide some objective information about detrusor and urethral function.

Where a habit problem is suspected from the history or a frequency/volume chart, explanation and retaining exercises, encouraging her to suppress the desire and hold her urine for increasingly longer periods is often successful, sometimes aided by anticholinergics.

If retention with overflow is present it may respond to urethral dilatation and subsequent cholinergic stimulants, but in many cases intermittent catheterisation is necessary.

With loss of awareness intermittent catheterisation may help but is less likely than with retention owing to the underlying problem. Long term indwelling catheters are poorly tolerated especially urethral catheters and for these ladies and those with unresponsive intractable detrusor problems or small capacity bladders as found with chronic interstitial cystitis, the help of the local continence adviser is invaluable. These advisers will be able to advise on the most appropriate appliances, garments, bed protection etc and offer practical help to the patients family and carers.

8. Ovarian cancer has a silent onset and an unfavourable outcome. How may the General Practitioner help with its early diagnosis and with the care of the patient with terminal disease.

A straightforward question designed to test your knowledge of the facilities available for terminal care. The first part of the question needs but a brief answer as there is very little one can do in the absence of a satisfactory screening test. The question is clear and it does not ask for a discussion on the pathology of ovarian cancer or its treatment. It may be tempting to write a page on those aspects especially as there is so little to say about its diagnosis. It may make you feel better but will not count for any marks and will tell the marker that you have either not read or not understood the question.

Key words: early diagnosis; care; terminal disease

Rough outline:

    diagnosis
    no screening procedure
    no early symptoms
    high index of suspicion with symptoms which might be related; abdominal swelling; distension; indigestion take every opportunity to exclude ovarian enlargement; smears; coil checks
    if mass found refer for confirmation and management

Management

    a) physical
        pain: analgesia; oral or subcutaneous infusion; pain clinics
        constipation
        urinary symptoms
        ascites

    b) emotional/social

        trusting relationship
        domiciliary care; social workers; Marie Curie/MacMillan nurses
        hospice care
        hospital care; community; DGH
        family support; bereavement counselling

Model answer:

Because of the characteristically silent nature of ovarian cancer and the lack of a screening procedure there is little one can do to make the diagnosis before there are signs or symptoms, by which time the condition is usually already well established. One should maintain a high index of suspicion and if a woman presents complaining of symptoms which could possibly be related the diagnosis should be excluded. Such symptoms are abdominal distension or a swelling, dyspareunia, lower abdominal discomfort and indigestion (a common finding for which there is often no obvious explanation).

One should take every opportunity also to exclude ovarian enlargement when performing pelvic examinations, e.g. when taking a smear, fitting or checking an IUCD, or when a woman presents with any gynaecological symptoms. If ovarian enlargement is suspected early referral to a specialist is indicated. Where the enlargement is less than 7 cm in diameter in a premenopausal woman it may be a functional cyst and it is permissible to re-examine her a month later to see if it has resolved. If the mass persists referral is indicated. Where there is a feeling of fullness in the adnexum but a definite mass cannot be felt the position can be clarified by ultrasound examination if local arrangements and facilities permit direct GP access.

The GP has a major role in the management of a terminally ill patient, both with the physical symptoms and with the emotional and social needs.

If the patient has pain it is essential to treat it adequately, starting with mild agents and increasing the potency and dose as required. Oral agents are appropriate initially and excellent results can be obtained even when opiates are necessary with morphine sulphate tablets, allowing the patient to remain ambulant. However, gastro-intestinal symptoms, exacerbated by the morphine may make parenteral therapy preferable. Battery driven portable syringe drivers allow satisfactory subcutaneous administration of diamorphine. Anti-emetics should be given wherever necessary and the dose of opiate can often be reduced by concurrent use of phenothiazines. Where pain is intractable the help of the local pain clinic should be sought, the Consultant could make a domiciliary visit if necessary.

Nausea should be treated with anti-emetics and constipation, often related to analgesia, should be watched for and treated promptly.

Urinary symptoms are variable; frequency or retention are not uncommon. If severe and incapacitating a catheter may provide relief.

Ascites can be troublesome and although surgical implantation of shunts can help one must remember that one is treating a person not a condition and in many cases paracentesis is appropriate to give, albeit temporary relief.

The emotional needs of terminally ill patients must not be under-estimated, this is the time they need the most support. The family doctor is in the best position to know the family and develop a trusting, caring relationship. The patient may or may not wish to know the true position and sensitive conversation should soon make this apparent. Encourage-ment of open communication and positive attitudes can be rewarding for all concerned.

The GPs knowledge of the family relationships, facilities and ability to cope will determine whether care should be at home, in a hospice or hospital (also depending on local facilities). Home care is often psycho-logically better for the patient and the support of the district nurse and specialist agencies such as the Macmillan nurses and Marie Curie nurses (who provide a night time service allowing the other members of the family to get some rest) make this possible. Social workers help with liaison with home help services and schools where young children are involved.

It may be that circumstances do not permit home care, or the family feel unable to cope with the emotional traumas. They also need support and must not be made to feel guilty. Hospice facilities, if available, provide care for the whole family in a pleasant environment and even when home care is intended it may be necessary to use hospice facilities either as a 'break' or in the final stages, thus the GP can introduce the idea and encourage the patient and family to familiarise themselves with the hospice and the staff at an early stage.

Sometimes it is necessary to utilise hospital facilities in the later stages. Where local community hospitals exist these are often less 'clinical' than DGHs and are more accessible for visiting by both family and GP.

Finally, the relatives must be assured of continuing care and support after the patient has died.

9. Discuss your investigation and management of a couple concerned with their inability to conceive and comment briefly on further investigation that may be necessary.

This is a question designed to test your approach to investigating infertility in the surgery. It is asking in very general terms for your approach. Do not waste time writing about treatment techniques beyond those you would use in the surgery. Writing about AID, IVF and GIFT in any detail is inappropriate. Because of the general nature of the question your answer will need to be general too. This can prove rather frustrating as it is impossible to write all you would like in the time. Be very careful not to overrun your time which is very easy to do with these very general questions.

Key words: your; investigation and management; couple; briefly; further investigation

Rough outline:

history
primary or secondary
previous relationships and any pregnancies
duration of infertility
previous contraception/any problems
frequency of intercourse/any problems
menstrual cycle
past medical history of both partners
male: sexually transmitted disease (STD) mumps, trauma, orchidopexy, hernia
female: STD, appendicitis, peritonitis, galactorrhoea, PID, any domestic or outside pressures?

Examination

male: general, testes, penis, varicocele, vasa
female: general, breasts, pelvic

Investigations

seminal analysis; ovulation: basal temperature chart (BTC)/ progesterone; tubal patency-hysterosalpingogram (HSG); laparoscopy; postcoital test (PCT)

Management

> of cause if found: ovulation induction/referral if tubal or male factor

> if no cause explanation reassurance, review
> ?referral/GIFT (gamete intrafallopian transfer)

Further investigation

> prolactin; thyroid function; FSH/LH; pituitary fossa
> X-ray

Model answer:

The most important step in the investigation of any couple presenting with infertility is to take a full history from both partners, separately as well as together as one partner may have some relevant details they may wish to withold from the other.

Details one would wish to elicit are whether they have had any previous pregnancies together or with any previous partner, how long they have been trying, any previous contraception (there may be post pill anovulation or if she has had an IUCD there may be a tubal problem). In order to assess whether they are giving themselves a fair chance the frequency of intercourse is important and whether they are trying to time intercourse in relation to the cycle, if so in what way. Any discomfort or difficulty with intercourse should be noted.

Details of her menstrual cycle may give clues to whether she is ovulating or not.

The past medical history of both partners is important. Has he had any history of testicular problems such as orchidopexy, herniorrhaphy as a child, trauma, orchitis, post pubertal mumps, or any sexually transmitted disease? Has she had a history of pelvic inflammatory disease, appendicitis, peritonitis or sexually transmitted disease (STD)? Has she noticed any galactorrhoea or any hirsutism?

Are there any pressures within the relationship, perhaps through the infertility, or within the family, or at work?

Following the history a clinical examination of both partners is desirable, this helps to underline that infertility is to be regarded as the problem of the couple rather than an individual. For the male a general examination should include particular note about any deformity of the penis, the size and consistency of the testes, the presence or absence of a varicocele and presence of the vasa. With the woman a general examination should include checking the breasts and a pelvic examination to exclude any masses.

Following this a number of investigations would be arranged to see if there is any detected problem with ovulation, tubal patency or any apparent male factor.

The male factor is checked by arranging for the local laboratory to examine a fresh semen sample, collected in the morning without any ejaculation the night before, directly into a clean container and delivered to the lab within one hour of production.

Ovulation is best confirmed by estimation of luteal phase serum progesterone levels taken one week before the anticipated onset of a period. Where the cycle is irregular samples should be taken on day 21 and then every week to menstruation. A basal temperature chart is less precise than progesterone levels and if used for more than 3 months can become a source of anxiety in itself.

Tubal patency can be tested by hysterosalpingography if the local X-ray department allows direct GP access for the investigation. Otherwise tubal patency testing would require referral, when laparoscopic examination may be chosen.

A postcoital test (PCT) allows examination of cervical mucus to see if the mucus is showing normal ovulatory changes and whether there are sperm present and if so if they are surviving. A PCT is best done just before the anticipated day of ovulation and the woman asked to come up in the morning having had intercourse the night before.

The management depends upon the detection of any underlying cause. Where there is a tubal problem referral is indicated to the local infertility service for consideration of tubal surgery, IVF or adoption. Male factors require referral for assessment, AID may be appropriate for some couples where there is azoospermia or severe oligospermia. Ovulation problems can often be treated in the surgery. If she is not ovulating estimation of prolactin, FSH and LH and thyroid function tests are appropriate. A raised prolactin in the presence of normal thyroid function needs further assessment of the pituitary with X-rays to exclude erosion of the bony margins of the pituitary fossa, and visual field checks. If normal bromocryptine therapy can be commenced. Abnormal thyroid function should be investigated and treated appropriately. A raised LH with reversal of the FSH/LH ratio by more than 3:1 may point to polycystic ovary syndrome. Testosterone levels should be checked and ovulation can be stimulated by Rehibin or clomiphene or tamoxifen therapy where the gonadotrophin levels are normal.

If no cause is found and they have been trying for over a year, having intercourse throughout the cycle on average two or more times a week, they are classed as 'unexplained' infertility. Referral to the local infertility service is appropriate with full details of the results of investigations performed. There is an increasing tendency for such couples to be offered the option of Gamete Intrafallopian Transfer (GIFT) as further in depth studies and in vitro sperm/mucus testing has not been found to improve the outlook.

It is important to bear in mind that even with new high technology techniques the chances of conception for couples with two years infertility is probably no more than one chance in three, therefore part of the overall management may well include long term counselling and support.

10. A 35 year old woman presents with a two year history of recurrent lower abdominal pain. Discuss the likely causes and appropriate investigations.

A clear question asking about a defined problem. Pay particular attention to the wording of the question.

Key words: 35 year old; two year history; recurrent; lower abdominal; likely; appropriate; investigations

Note that you are not asked for management, however, a therapeutic trial of treatment may be appropriate and should be discussed briefly.

Rough outline:

> detailed history; what is the pattern; ?cyclical; related to periods?; related to bowel action?; related to intercourse?; related to micturition?; nature of pain; duration; radiation; aggravating and relieving factors; any domestic or work stresses?

> likely causes: irritable bowel syndrome (IBS); endometriosis: pelvic inflammatory disease (PID); dysmen; stress

> investigations: examination; swabs; laparoscopy; therapeutic trial of treatment; barium studies: sigmoidoscopy/colonoscopy.

Model answer:

There are a number of conditions which may present with recurrent lower abdominal pain. The most likely in a woman of this age include Irritable Bowel Syndrome (IBS) which is now very common as a result of the low fibre content of the average diet today with a high proportion of refined foods. Endometriosis and pelvic inflammatory disease are likely to be associated with other gynaecological symptoms (dyspareunia or dysmenorrhoea) or findings. Primary dysmenorrhoea is unlikely at this age.

Chronic urinary problems are unlikely to present primarily as recurrent pain especially in this age group, although lower abdominal pain may be a feature of chronic trigonitis. Ureteric colic, although usually described as radiating from the loin, might present within the very broad compass of lower abdominal pain.

A full history and careful examination will often point to the most likely

65

cause, although it can be very difficult to differentiate a gynaecological cause from a bowel problem.

A detailed history is essential paying particular attention to the pattern of recurrence, whether it is daily, or cyclical in relation to her periods or whether the recurrence is random. The presence of any aggravating factors should be sought such as intercourse, menstruation, defaecation or micturition. The nature of the pain, its site, radiation and duration together with any relieving factors are important. It is not uncommon to find that abdominal pains are perceived to be worse in the presence of stressful factors either at home or work and these should be enquired about.

Any previous history of similar pain should be sought. A full review of systems must be made.

Clinical examination must include abdominal palpation determining the site of the pain and the presence of any tenderness, guarding or rebound. Pelvic examination should detect any apparent gynaecological problem. A fixed retroverted uterus with nodularity in the pouch of Douglas (POD) may reflect endometriosis or pelvic adhesions. If there is any pelvic tenderness careful attention should be paid to its site. If lateral or posterior it may well be associated with the bowel. Palpation of the urethra and over the trigone will reveal tenderness suggestive of a urinary cause.

If it is thought that pelvic inflammatory disease is the cause then cervical swabs can be taken looking for chlamydia in addition to the usual organisms and antibiotic therapy commenced using a broad spectrum agent which will cover chlamydia such as erythromycin or doxycycline and an agent to cover anaerobes such as metronidazole. If endometriosis is thought possible referral is appropriate for consideration of a laparoscopy. Many cases are due to IBS and where this is thought to be the case a therapeutic trial is appropriate. In the long term, dietary reeducation is needed to have a high fibre intake. In the short term this can be mimicked by giving a bulking agent such as Fybogel or Regulan and an anti-spasmodic such as colofac.

If a urinary cause is considered a mid stream specimen of urine should be examined. Urinary problems presenting as recurrent pain in a woman of 35 are unusual and referral would be appropriate.

Where a therapeutic trial has been unsuccessful for either suspected PID or IBS then referral is indicated either to the gynaecologist who will probably offer a laparoscopy or, where a bowel cause is considered most likely, to a gastroenterological unit which may undertake fibreoptic colonoscopy. Where the symptoms are accompanied by a change in bowel habit, early referral is indicated.

SAMPLE ESSAY QUESTIONS: FAMILY PLANNING

11. Discuss the counselling of a young married woman who requests a sterilisation operation.

A broad question which allows you to demonstrate your knowledge of family planning and your views of the role of sterilisation in particular. It should be possible to complete your answer comfortably within the 45 minute allocation.

Key words: young; married; sterilisation

Rough outline:

Why is she asking?

> parity, financial hardship; contraceptive difficulty; as a bid to save an unstable marriage; inability to cope with domestic pressures?

Why has she come alone?

> does husband know of her request; does he agree with it; is he apathetic or regards it as her responsibility?

Relevant details:

> age, parity; ages of children; current contraception and reason for wish to change; previous contraception and any problems; awareness of alternative forms of contraception, duration and stability of marriage; awareness of irreversibility of the operation and its inherent failure rate. Past history of hypertension, thromboembolic disease, abdominal surgery, anaesthetic difficulties. ·

Examination:

> general including obesity, blood pressure, vaginal to exclude pathology and take smear if appropriate

Each case should be judged on its own merit rather than be arbitrary rules. Postpone decision if youngest child is less than 6 months old because of risk of Sudden Infant Death Syndrome, or if relationship is unstable.

Model answer:

When approached by this lady one would wish to know why she wants to be sterilised, to determine whether it is a considered decision reached after consideration of alternatives and all the implications of the operation, or if it is an impulsive request based on a reaction to the stresses of a young family, financial hardships, perhaps an attempt to save an unstable relationship or reluctance to comply with contraceptive techniques. To this end one should ascertain:

> her age
> her parity, with the ages of the children
> the duration of the marriage and its stability (previous marital history of the partners may be relevant)
>
> any domestic pressures
> present contraceptive technique and her reason for wanting to change
> previous contraceptive techniques and any problems experienced
> her awareness of alternative forms of contraception her menstrual history, as proven menorrhagia may merit consideration of hyster-ectomy as the method of choice.

If it appears to be an impulsive decision she should be encouraged to discuss the underlying problem(s) and try to get her to see them from a broader perspective, explaining that sterilisation is meant to be a permanent measure and that she would thus be unable to change her mind later if there were a change in circumstance, such as improved financial situation, breakdown of relationship and subsequent re-marriage, loss of partner or loss of a child.

Potentially suitable alternative forms of contraception should be discussed with her.

The role of the doctor in this situation is that of counselling and advising what is considered to be most appropriate in the circumstances rather than simply being a referral source.

Each request should be looked at on its own merit rather than following rigid rules of age and parity.

If her request is thought inappropriate she should be told explaining the reasons and advising what is thought most appropriate. If she persisted with the request the matter should be discussed with her and her husband together, and if they then still felt they wanted a sterilisation, referral to a specialist explaining my opinion in the referral letter would be appropriate.

If her request was thought appropriate she should be reminded of the irreversible nature and inherent failure rate of up to 5 cases per thousand depending upon the technique. The question of which partner should have the operation should be discussed – have they considered the pros and cons of vasectomy, would the husband agree to consider vasectomy? Are there any medical reasons for recommending vasectomy?

Where there is a history of menorrhagia, especially where there has been a fall in haemoglobin level it is important to document this and to determine if there is uterine pathology as this may influence the gynaecologist to discuss the possible role of hysterectomy.

A sterilisation is rarely a life saving procedure and one should do everything possible to minimise the risks of operation. Thus the obese should lose weight, smokers be encouraged to stop etc. A smear should be taken if she has not had a normal smear within the past 3 years.

Where there is a significant past medical history, or where the woman is very obese or an inveterate smoker her husband should be strongly recommended to have a vasectomy.

If vasectomy is acceptable the procedure should be discussed explaining the need for continuing contraception until the seminal analyses confirm azoospermia.

If their youngest child is under 6 months of age it is advisable for them to continue with present contraception until the child is beyond the small risk of Sudden Infant Death Syndrome.

In considering where to refer appropriate requests local waiting lists would be relevant as the couple may wish for referral outside the NHS if the waiting list is long. However a wait of say 3 months does allow for further reflection in light of full knowledge of the implications of the procedure. It is not uncommon for women on waiting lists to change their mind and it is too late once the operation has been performed.

12. A patient requests that you fit an intrauterine contraceptive device. Discuss the advantages and disadvantages of this form of contraception and describe how you would assess its suitability in a particular case.

The first sentence of this question is irrelevant to your answer. The first part of the question is simply factual and brief. The second assesses your knowledge of contraceptive techniques and in particular what you consider the role of an IUCD to be. This need not be a drawn out answer and you should finish the question comfortably in the time allowed. You must state how you would assess a particular case, although this will be in general terms as the question does not define any details of a 'particular' case.

Key words: discuss; advantages and disadvantages; you

Rough outline:

advantages
> ease of compliance
> minimal inconvenience of 2–3 years changes
> reliability
> no interference with spontaneity of sex life
> easily reversed

disadvantages
> increased menstrual loss
> dysmenorrhoea
> increased risk of pelvic inflammatory disease (PID)/sepsis
> risk of expulsion
> no protection against STD
> failure rate

assessment
> why does she want an IUCD?
> previous contraception and any problems
> current contraception and any problems
> parity
> ability to cope with alternative methods requiring greater compliance
> ?past history of PID
> ?past history of ectopic
> menstrual history
> past medical history
> size of uterus/fibroids?

any vaginitis
normal smear?

Model answer:

An intrauterine contraceptive device is for many women an ideal form of contraception. Once fitted it need only be changed every two to three years (if an inert, non-copper device it can be left indefinitely). It does not require any compliance as is required with oral agents and barrier methods and does not interfere with spontaneity as do the barrier methods. It is easily removed with immediate return of fertility.

However, it does have some drawbacks. The presence of a foreign body in the uterus may lead to increased menstrual loss, dysmenorrhoea and an increased incidence of pelvic infection. It can also be expelled, particularly in the first period after insertion, thus occasional checks that the strings are visible is advisable. It has been said that ectopic pregnancies are more common. This is not true, in fact the actual incidence of ectopics is actually reduced, but of the pregnancies occurring in women with a coil in situ up to one in 25 is an ectopic, thus creating the illusion of an increased incidence. IUCDs do not offer any protection against sexually transmitted diseases.

In assessing its suitability in a particular case I would determine why the woman was asking for a coil. Details of her present and past contraception and any problems are relevant. She may find that she forgets to take her pills regularly or has conceived following failure of a barrier method. There may be a medical history which contraindicates the use of a combined oral preparation such as deep vein thrombosis (DVT), or cholestatic jaundice. A past history of pelvic inflammatory disease (PID) or ectopic pregnancy would tend to influence me away from recommending its use. When discussing a patients suitability for a coil she must be aware of the relative failure rate of this form of contraception.

Her parity is important; because of the risk of pelvic infection and subsequent infertility. One tends to be more hesitant in fitting IUCDs in nulliparous women although specially designed small devices are available. Her ability to comply with alternative methods will be an important consideration.

Her age should be considered, for instance in women approaching the menopause a barrier method may offer sufficient protection. In view of the tendency to heavier periods details of her menstrual history are important and estimation of her full blood count indices if she feels her loss is heavy.

Her plans for future pregnancies should be discussed because if her family is complete, sterilisation of either partner may be an appropriate option not previously considered.

On examination the size and shape of the uterus are important as distortion from fibroids or congenital anomalies are relative contra-indications to its use. I would also check for any masses or tenderness which may suggest pelvic infection. If there is any sign of vaginitis swabs would be sent for bacteriological examination and if she had not had a smear in the past 3 years I would take one.

Having taken a history and examined her I would consider the overall picture and discuss what I felt were appropriate alternatives as she may not be aware of the range of methods available. If there were no contraindications and after informed consideration of the alternatives, the advantages and disadvantages of an IUCD, I would agree to her request. If I felt that there were definite contraindications I would explain my reasons and decline her request and offer her what I consider to be the most appropriate alternatives. If she still wished to have a device fitted she would be free to seek a second opinion at the family planning clinic.

3. THE CLINICAL EXAMINATION

In this part of the DRCOG exam you need to convince the examiner that you are competent to diagnose and manage the patient's condition. Attention to detail is important.

As this exam is very practical in its emphasis you should get as much practice as possible in examining patients and presenting cases. Ask your consultant or registrar for their help as it is often the simple basic principles of examination which lead to a candidate's downfall. However, do not get dispirited in these practice sessions if the 'examiner' is over critical as it *is* important that you develop the correct technique of examination and presentation.

Whilst not wishing to appear restrictive please remember that medicine is a conservative profession. Both patients and other members of the profession expect a certain standard of dress and demeanour of doctors. Avoid flashy clothes: for men there is much to commend the quiet dark suit, white shirt, medical school tie and polished shoes – the ubiquitous interview, exam and courtroom attire! Women should wear a conservative dress or suit. A neat, well groomed appearance is likely to meet with a favourable response from the examiner. If you wish to wear a white coat it is quite acceptable but is not compulsory.

There is considerable scope for preparation in this section of the examination. Most examinees will have taken histories from and examined numerous women during the course of their work. However, in the exam situation one should strive for perfection considering all aspects of the history from physical, psychological and social view points. Practise only makes perfect when it is structured to ensure all areas are covered and nothing is missed. In devising such a structure it is useful to consider the information available to the examiners during the exam; they will have cards with details of the key points of the case on them which act as prompts for further questions. Although the notes are available, the examiners will not necessarily be aware of all the intimate details. This can become a major advantage to the candidate.

You will usually be shown to your allotted patient (who may be an obstetric, gynaecological or family planning patient) by a sympathetic Registrar or Sister. Identify yourself to the patient in a friendly and confident manner and remember that the patient is attending the examination as a favour to you and the examiners, so treat her accordingly. Most patients know the score and try to be helpful, but a dithering anxious approach will not impress them.

You have 20 minutes in which to take the history and perform such general and abdominal examination as you think appropriate. You should *not* perform a vaginal examination unless the examiner is with you. Make notes on the paper provided as no-one expects you to memorise all the details. Whilst allowing the patient to tell her own story, remember that time is limited and specific direct questions are often required, it helps when introducing yourself to the patient to tell her what you require from her, e.g. "Hello, my name is Richard. I would like to spend 10 minutes asking you some questions about your condition and then spend 5 minutes examining you, is that alright?"

Having established a rapport with the patient ask her what her problem is and what her doctors have told her, including the diagnosis but beware that she may unwittingly deceive you.

Use your eyes. If there is a urine sample, it is there for a reason, test it. Conversely, if there is no specimen and an obstetric patient has hypertension you can use this to advantage when presenting the case by slipping in 'unfortunately there was no urine available for testing'.

Before the examiners arrive run through the main features of the case with the patient to make sure you have got things clear, underline the important details both positive and negative.

When the examiners arrive be courteous and confident, whilst acknowledging that they are in control of the proceedings. You have 20 minutes with the examiners.

After the introductory formalities the examiner will begin his questioning. Listen carefully to what he asks and only answer what is asked, not what you think he wants. He will vary his approach from candidate to candidate to prevent tedium.

Common opening questions include:
"Would you present the case", or "Tell me about this case".

These are straightforward, but be prepared for such requests as:
"Tell me what conclusions you have come to".
"What differential diagnoses have you considered?"

"What treatment would you advise?"
"How would you manage the case?"

These openers negate your full presentation, so be prepared for quick changes in your line of thought.

When the examiner proceeds to specific questions, make sure you understand what is being asked for. Think before answering, and answer only the question asked. Do not volunteer additional information unless you are certain of your ground and can answer further questions on the subject. Experienced examiners have a knack of picking up these additional details offered by candidates and pursuing them, thus ensuring that the unwary dig themselves into an inextricably large pit!

You will be asked to repeat the abdominal examination and to perform a vaginal examination in cases where the examiners consider it appropriate. The examiners may also ask you to demonstrate some physical signs you have elicited. Before demonstrating what you have been asked, reassure the patient by explaining what you are going to do. This applies particularly if asked to perform a pelvic examination. You must not on any account hurt or upset the patient when examining her. If you do you will be heavily penalised.

When you have concluded the examination, cover the patient with the sheet. The patient will appreciate this and you will 'score' with the examiner. Do not forget to wash your hands after a pelvic examination, the examiner will be observing. (It also takes a little time out of the allocation, and every little helps!)

Obstetric clinical presentation schedule

Key points
Introduce the patient to the examiners and vice versa.

Introduction
Have a standard format which is brief and to the point e.g. Mrs X is 35 years old and is now 34 weeks advanced in her 4th pregnancy.

Summarise the main features of the history.
This is only a list. It should hopefully be identical to the list that the examiners have in front of them.

e.g. The main features are:

1. Hypertensive disease of pregnancy ⎫
2. Intrauterine growth retardation ⎭ in relation to this pregnancy

3. Previous stillbirth (in relation to previous pregnancy)

4. Single parent family (social features)

5. Positive family history of hypertension (family features)

Do not elaborate at this stage as it will lead to confusion and may wake the examiners up!

Details of this pregnancy

Start at the beginning and work through as if unfolding a story in a logical progression. Don't let the examiners interrupt if possible.

1. Planned or unplanned
       prior contraception/failure of contraception
       prepregnancy counselling

2. Gestational assessment
       LMP – date + certainty
           – cycle length + regularity
           – prior contraception
           – bleeding after LMP
       EDC – from this date

       Ultrasound scan at 16 weeks
           – confirms dates or not
           – by this scan is now X weeks and EDC is Y

3. Care plan
       booking arrangements, GP/hospital
       antenatal care – shared ⎫
                   – GP unit ⎬ Try and look at the
                   – hospital only ⎭ antenatal card
                   – (physician involved)
                   – preparation classes
                   – birth plan or not
                   – breast feeding or not

4. This pregnancy was normal until X weeks. .
> Then elaborate on main features listed previously giving details of symptoms and management plan, with respect to likely mode and timing of delivery.

Obstetric history
> List the prior pregnancies and their outcome.
>> – the year
>> – antenatal problems
>> – mode of delivery
>> – postnatal problems
>> – outcome – birth weight
>>>> – name
>>>> – condition at birth and feeding
>>>> – present health

Gynaecology history
> Give date and result of last smear (often forgotten)

Medical history
Surgical history } relate to main features
Psychiatric history

Drug history
> Including iron and folic acid tabs.

Allergies

Social history
> This is the most important part. The examiners will not be aware of the details! So tell them.

> Think – how does the pregnancy affect her and the family's social conditions?
> – how do the social conditions affect the pregnancy?

> marital status
> occupation – future plans
> – maternity leave or not?
> – will she return?
> – who will look after the baby?
> finances – will the pregnancy affect them?
> housing – is there room in the house?

husband   – paternity leave
              – family support
If in-patient – who is looking after the children?
              – are they visiting?
smoking status
alcohol consumption (units)

Future plans after delivery
contraception plans
postnatal follow up
preconception clinic next pregnancy
immunisation plans for the baby

Conclude history with summary of main findings

After presentation of the history, the examiners may ask for the main findings on examination of the woman. They usually ask you to demonstrate your findings. Again, stay calm and make it look as though you do this every day - which you do. It is helpful to develop a style so that you omit nothing. Here are some key points to help:

Key points

– The woman you are examining is a human being and should be treated with respect.

– Ask her for permission to examine her.

– Correct positioning is essential. She should be lying flat with 1 or 2 pillows. Ask if she is comfortable lying on her back as many pregnant women are not because of caval compression.

– Do not expose the woman unduly. Her abdomen should be adequately exposed but use the blankets sensibly.

During inspection, from the end of the bed it helps the examiners if you tell them what you see. They may interrupt your train of thought if you don't. Remember to look for operation scars. Laparoscopy scars are easily missed. Make confident but brief statements. If you say that "there is an abdominal swelling consistent with pregnancy" the examiners may well reply with "tell me why?" So be prepared. Only visible fetal movements enable one to state that the swelling is a gravid uterus.

– Always ask the woman if her abdomen is tender before you touch her. If you are seen to inflict pain then you will fail.

– If you use a tape measure to assess fundal height, then be confident in its use.

– Look for ankle oedema by pressing over the lower anterior tibia gently.

– Check the blood pressure, with the woman sitting on the edge of the bed. Caval compression will alter the reading.

– Always ask to check the urine for sugar and protein.

– Restore the woman back to her previous state. Remember to ask her if anything you have discussed has worried her and if she has any questions. This will impress the examiners no end.

Having concluded the presentation and examination the examiners will whisk you off to discuss the management of the case away from the patient. They may also diverge from the topic and ask other questions. You may well be shown CTGs or a partogram. Try and work logically through the problems using the frameworks discussed in the next chapter.

NB. A similar schedule can be designed for a gynaecological or family planning case. Try and design one you are happy with.

Common errors in the clinical examination

As all DRCOG candidates have completed a 6 month approved post in the specialty of obstetrics and gynaecology, it is expected that they will be familiar with obstetric and gynaecological history taking. This expectation is, on occasions, often ill founded. The examination often determines marked weaknesses in the candidate's ability to elicit relevant information and present it concisely. Good application of basic principles and good technique are the key to success in a clinical examination.

Common errors in history taking include monotonous 'Dalek-toned' presentations with incorrect emphasis on clinical facts. In obstetric cases it is mandatory to state the first day of the last menstrual period and hence the expected date of confinement. Equally important is to convey to the examiner that the patient's present gestation is not in doubt, determined by the fact that her cycle is regular, there is no recent history of oral contraception and that at 16–18 weeks the dates were confirmed by ultrasound scan. Regrettably these facts are not stated clearly enough when the candidate presents them. Without accurate knowledge of the patient's dates, meaningful ante-natal assessment cannot take place. The candidate must emphasise his awareness of this point to the examiners.

The exact order in which the candidate presents the facts is best left to the individual. At some point in an obstetric case it is essential to mention the details of when the patient 'booked' at the hospital (first attended in pregnancy). This fact is, again, sadly neglected in a fair proportion of examinees. The 'Booking' time and 'findings' will give you, and the examiner, a guide to the condition of the patient earlier in the pregnancy. For example, in a hypertensive patient at 36 weeks, it is invaluable to determine the patient was normotensive when she was first seen. The 'Booking' details should be mentioned in the history of the present pregnancy. It is unlikely that there would be any abnormal findings if the patient subsequently had shared care with her General Practitioner, and this point should be emphasised during the course of the history.

In gynaecological cases, details of the patient's menstrual cycle, duration of bleeding, frequency of cycle along with the date of the last period are mandatory. Irregular bleeding, post coital or inter-menstrual bleeding, should similarly be noted and emphasised. Some mention of the patient's current contraception and sexual problems should also be determined. These points are often omitted, and are an essential part of the history and subsequent management of the case. For example, it is important to know if a patient with a prolapse is sexually active or not – over zealous repairs may result in subsequent dyspareunia or apareunia. Facts regarding the sexual history are often omitted because of examination nerves or embarrassment.

At the end of the presentation, in haste to finish the history, candidates frequently continue to detail their examination findings. It is sensible to pause and regain composure. A short summary of the history is particularly useful here, and ensures that the examiners have noted that you have satisfactorily elicited the salient points. Do *not* make the mistake (as many do) of re-presenting the history almost in its entirety, for then it will not be a summary, as a summary, by definition, must be *concise*.

Errors in the examination of the patient during the clinical are frequent. The common mistakes again usually reflect poor technique, as well as poor clinical practice. Failure to examine breasts and enquire about intended breast feeding is extremely common. "No chaperone" is an occasional excuse offered by the male candidate. "Sort of" is another reply which is even more unacceptable. "I had a quick look when listening to the chest" does not inspire confidence or suggest clinical honesty.

Incorrect assessment of blood pressure and oedema are frequently encountered. The blood pressure is often taken during pregnancy in the supine position, neglecting the fact that the gravid uterus would produce supine hypotension. Similarly, oedema is assessed by compressing the medial malleolus instead of applying digital pressure to the anterior surface of the tibia. Again, candidates often check for oedema in one leg, assuming it will be the same in the other. Beware of the silent deep venous thrombosis, or orthopaedic conditions affecting one leg.

Most mistakes in the 'clinical' occur during the abdominal examination. Inspection of the abdomen is often inadequate with failure to mention pigmentation, striae and operation scars. The error is compounded if the candidate has earlier mentioned in the history that the patient has had a previous surgery, such as a Caesarean section, and then neglects to comment on the scar during the examination.

Deficiencies in abdominal palpation probably constitute the most errors. When this is coupled with bad technique, disaster is inevitable. It is, therefore, mandatory to have a rehearsed or set order of presentation. For example, the uterine size is consistent with so many weeks of pregnancy as determined by the fundal height and the girth measurement. The uterus contains a single fetus, longitudinal lie, cephalic presentation, the number of fifths of the head palpable should be commented on and whether or not the head is engaged. The fetal back, and the side of the fetal back, should also be noted and whether the fetal heart is heard and regular. Additional comment regarding amniotic fluid volume and fetal movement will also impress the examiner, particularly in cases of polyhydramnios, or 'small for dates' cases.

Less impressive are remarks that 'the head is engaging' or 'the head is fixed and must therefore be engaged'. The head is either engaged or not, determined by the number of the fifths of the head palpable per abdomen. i.e. if two fifths, or less, are palpable then the head is engaged. Attempts to auscultate the fetal heart on the opposite side of the fetal back similarly suggest weakness in the examination technique, and often un-nerve the candidate who becomes aware that the examiners know that he, or she, is not listening to the fetal heart at the right site.

The cardinal sin in clinical examination, which fortunately is not encountered so often, is dishonesty. Manufacturing physical signs to fit the expected picture is totally unacceptable. If you are uncertain of the presenting part (in an obstetric examination) it is much better to say so, rather than stating it is a breech presentation because the patient has previously told you so. Similarly 'hearing' a heart murmur, which is not there, because a patient is suspected of cardiac disease will not look impressive and it will be heavily penalised. *You must say what you find, not what you expect to find.* In this situation at the very worst you are only guilty of missing a clinical sign. To be guilty of this *and* clinical dishonesty will be penalised most severely.

The candidates who are clear, concise and show good clinical acumen are those that pass with least difficulty. The examiners are human and do understand that candidates will be nervous and take this into consideration. The more difficult the case, often the more sympathetic, and considerate, the examiners. Remember this and, therefore, do not panic if your case appears complex and that you are struggling to cope with it.

4. THE ORAL EXAMINATION

This is usually the last hurdle and is regarded by many as the most awesome. The candidate often feels vulnerable and can easily be intimidated by the setting. A polite manner is always expected and specific points such as standing until invited to take a seat at the beginning and offering your thanks at the end of the examination will do no harm. Attention to dress and appearance are just as important as for the clinical.

You will be confronted by two examiners and a variety of torture implements for 20 minutes. It is likely that there will be twenty or so other candidates in the room at the same time, each with two examiners. This adds up to a lack of privacy as you are separated only by screens, with background noise making concentration very difficult. It is essential to try to remain calm and actively generate a positive attitude to the event. The examiners are only human (usually) and they are trying to pass you. Remember you are being compared with your peers and not with them!

During your 20 minutes with the examiners the questions asked will cover aspects of obstetrics, gynaecology and family planning. In addition to straightforward questions, you may be asked to identify and discuss various items such as X-rays, laboratory reports, pathology specimens, CTG tracings, forceps, contraceptive items and common gynaecological instruments etc. Use your eyes. Think carefully before answering each question and avoid saying the first thing that comes into your head. If you answer without thinking you will get into trouble.

The examiner will usually pass from topic to topic, especially if you appear to know about a particular subject; this allows him to assess the breadth of your knowledge although you may find this very frustrating.

As in the clinical examination, only answer what is asked unless you are trying to lead the examiner along a definite path. You will undoubtedly benefit from some 'mock' oral sessions so ask your consultant and registrar for their help.

The examiners will start with an opening question and then gradually wind up the pressure until your limit is reached and this can feel frightening as your uncertainty increases during the questioning. This is however designed to assess your knowledge and skills. Don't be surprised by their lack of response to your answers they will be listening and often make notes to help them, which can become distracting. Try not to get paranoid. The end of the battle is marked by a bell and the ordeal will be over.

In such situations when the adrenaline is high it is easy to make mistakes and dig holes for yourself. This is not through lack of knowledge for most of us, but because of the way the information is presented to the examiner, leaving yourself open to their wrath. The knowledge you have should be assimilated in such a way that automatic recall can operate. The use of a check list early in revision will help you. However, knowledge is useless unless you present it well.

Most of the questions asked can be categorised into one of three main areas.

1. **Management questions**
    e.g. How would you manage a breech presentation at 36 weeks gestation?
2. **Factual knowledge questions**
    e.g. What are the causes of menorrhagia?
3. **Dilemmas and difficult problems**
    e.g. A fifteen year old girl asked you for the oral contraceptive pill. How would you deal with this?

Let us consider ways of answering these 3 different types of questions under exam conditions. It is essential to start at the beginning of your answer rather than half way through so that the examiner can see that your thought pattern is logical. To do this you need a *framework* on which to hang your answer. Let us look at the framework for each of these three areas.

1. **MANAGEMENT QUESTIONS:** These can often be daunting on the surface. However, with a little structure things become easy as we can relate the answer to our day to day experiences.

    A. **definition of problem**

    B. **assessment** (the collecting of information)

    | History | – key points |
    | Examination | – general, abdominal and pelvic |
    | Investigations | – urine tests |
    | | blood tests |

ultrasound and X-ray
cardiotocograph (CTG)
fetal monitoring

C. **planning**

Discuss the options available e.g.
GP continues treatment or referral of patient to the:
- Hospital unit
- Midwife
- Family planning clinic
- Health Visitors
- Social Services
- Self help groups

General advice for patient
Drug treatment
Surgical treatment
Remember to involve the patient in the decision and explain the likely outcomes.

D. **implementation of treatment**

E. **review**

Follow up is frequently used in general practice. However, it is often forgotten in exams. Remember it is useful for audit of the event in the future.

Now use this format to try and compile a watertight answer in response to the breech presentation at 36 weeks. You should find it helps.

2. FACTUAL KNOWLEDGE QUESTIONS: We all know the facts somewhere inside our heads but under stress one can never remember. Here are some frameworks that often help here.

A. **physical**
   psychological } these two areas are often forgotten
   social

B. **anatomical breakdown**

Local causes –	Gynaecological	Obstetric
	Vulval	Baby/Fetus
	Vaginal	Amniotic fluid
	Cervical	Placenta and Cord
	Uterine	Uterine wall
	Fallopian tube	Outside the uterus
	Ovarian	

General causes – (surgical sieve)
Congenital/Acquired

Endocrine	Hypothalamic
	Pituitary axis
	Sex hormones
Metabolic	Thyroid problems
	Diabetes

Pregnancy related
Infective	Acute
	Chronic

Inflammatory
Neoplasia + tumours
      – Benign
      – Malignant:Primary
                  Secondary
Vascular
Trauma
Iatrogenic
Nutritional
Idiopathic

3. DILEMMAS AND DIFFICULT PROBLEMS: Questions are often asked that appear complex and pose a series of dilemmas to the doctor involved, as in the example given. It is often difficult to know where to begin here. It helps to reflect the statement back to the examiners stating the dilemmas involved.

e.g. Giving advice to a 15 year old girl about the pill can be difficult. The problems and dilemmas are:

1.   Is it ethically and morally acceptable to prescribe the oral contraceptive pill to a minor (in the eyes of the law)? Is the doctor in effect giving her permission to have underage intercourse?

2. What is the legal position?

3. How will her parents react and do they have the right to know? Is there a conflict between confidentiality and the future doctor patient relationship?

4. Will she be able to comply with the technicalities of taking the combined pill?

5. Is there a hidden agenda in the presentation?
    i.e. Is asking for the pill her way of saying "I think I'm pregnant"?

6. What are the medical implications of starting young females on the oral contraceptive pill? And so on (there are many more).

Once the dilemma has been raised, one can set about discussing the options available. The examiners do not want a blinkered view point, so it helps to discuss the advantages and disadvantages of each option. Remember who is involved when dilemmas are raised.

1. The doctor, partners, hospital, midwife, nurse, health visitor, primary health care team

2. The patient, family and partner

3. The community at large

The costs and benefits of each option can be stated in relation to each group. You should end the answer with a decision saying why you feel it is the best option.

Always remember to (i.e. show the examiners that you would):

Explore the patients – Ideas
                      – Concerns
                      – Expectations

Use your skills of   – Active listening
                     – Reflecting
                     – Summarising
                     – Collecting important information
                     – Empathising
                     – Giving the patient time

It is hoped that by using these frameworks on which to hang your ideas each topic will be fully covered and the examiners will be aware of your logical thought processes. This technique is useful in any professional situation - not just in examinations!

THE MARKING SYSTEM

The clinical and oral examinations are each marked out of 100 points within a range of 47–53.

A mark of 53 indicates an excellent performance.
A mark of 52 indicates a good pass.
A mark of 51 indicates a pass at postgraduate level.
A mark of 50 indicates a borderline situation.
A mark of 49 is a fail but the examiners may be asked if they would be prepared to raise the mark at the examiners' meeting where all parts of the examination are considered.
A mark of 48 indicates a poor candidate.
A mark of 47 is an absolute failure. Candidates awarded 47 in the clinical will fail the examination irrespective of the overall mark obtained.

The clinical and oral marks are added to the mark for the written paper and the total mark is assessed. Candidates with 152 marks or more will pass providing they have passed in at least two components of the examination and have not been awarded 47 in the clinical. Candidates with 151 may pass if their lowest mark is 49 in the clinical or oral (with marks of 51 in the other two sections) and the examiners awarding that mark are prepared to raise the mark at the examiners' meeting.

5. GENERAL PRACTICE OBSTETRICS

1. THE DOCTORS BAG

The GP who provides maternity care for the practice population should carry the necessary equipment to deal with an emergency situation arising antenatally, during delivery and postnatally. It is important that the bag has adequate storage capacity and the equipment is accurately labelled and reviewed regularly. Emergency situations are always stressful for both the family and the doctor. Such problems for the doctor can be reduced by being prepared before the event has occurred.

Essentials:

      Sphygmomanometer
      Stethoscope
      Ophthalmoscope
      Torch
      Disposable gloves + obstetric cream + disposable speculum
      Urine testing equipment – clinistix – albustix
      Blood glucose testing strips
      BNF or MIMS
      Local phone numbers – ambulance
                               – hospitals
                                 – delivery suites and flying squad
                                    contact point
                                 – social services
                                 – partners home numbers
      Stationery   – Prescription pad (FP10)
                                 – Forms – temporary resident forms (FP19)
                                          – emergency treatment forms
                                          – blood forms
                                          – ultrasound forms
                                          – sick notes (FM3/FM5)

Resuscitation equipment:

      Tourniquet
      Micropore tape
      Scissors + Spencer Wells forceps
      IV cannulae

Syringes + needles
Blood bottles – FBC
            – Group and cross match
Giving sets   – N. saline
Swabs
Space blanket– for baby
Airways   – Brook
            – Neonatal airway
Mucus extractor
Endotracheal tubes   } Adult and
Laryngoscopes   } neonatal
Suturing equipment

Drugs:

The following can be recommended:
     Diazepam
     Diamorphine
     Syntocinon
     Ergometrine
     Syntometrine
     Hydralazine
     Dextrose 50%
     1% lignocaine for local anaesthesia
     Vitamin K_1
     Antiemetic e.g. Metoclopramide
     Water for injections
     Antiseptic wash

All drugs should be adequately labelled with batch number and expiry date. The doctor should regularly review his drugs and any used should be noted with the patients name and drug batch number.

Further reading:

A Guide to General Practice. The Oxford GP Group. 2nd 1987 edition. Blackwell Scientific.
Learning General Practice. J. Sandars and R. Baron. 1988 Pastest.

2. GP OBSTETRICS

Since 1970 there has been a progressive decline in the number of deliveries for which GPs and community midwives have been responsible. It can be assumed that the reason for the fall is that GP obstetrics is high risk but in several studies comparing the perinatal mortality rates for planned deliveries under the care of GPs and those under consultant care, results were equally good. In the analysis of the British Births Survey of 1970, the perinatal mortality rate was lower for women delivering under GP care at all levels of risk, except for the highest. Similar results were obtained from a study in New Zealand. Like all epidemiological studies, criticism can be made of the methodology, but a large review of GP obstetrics concluded that the case could not be proved either way 'there is no evidence to support the claim that the safest policy is for all women to give birth in hospital' (Campbell R MacFarlane. Where to be born? The Debate and the Evidence, Oxford. National Perinatal Epidemiology Unit 1987).

If the perinatal mortality rate is no longer a useful guide to policy, then morbidity and consumer satisfaction are more important. A recent study was done in the John Radcliffe Hospital, Oxford to compare women's reactions to consultant and general practitioner care (Klein M, Elbourne D, Lloyd I. Booking for Maternity Care – A Comparison of two Systems. Occasional Paper 31. Royal College of General Practitioners 1985).

In this study carefully matched cohorts of low risk women booked for either consultant (shared) care or general practitioner (community) care in the same hospital were compared. There were no significant differences in perinatal mortality between the groups. Interventions, such as induction, acceleration, episiotomy, analgesic drugs, regional anaesthesia, forceps delivery and intubation of the neonate occurred significantly less often in the community group. Women in the community group were seen by fewer medical and midwifery staff during labour and they were more likely to recognise those they did see. The community group found antenatal visits helpful and enjoyable, but there was no difference between the two groups in their experience during labour.

The provision of GP units allows patients to be offered a real choice, so important in the present climate of patient autonomy. However, in 1982 only 3.4% of births were in GP Units.

Preconceptional care

The aims of preconceptional care are to ensure:

93

a)   Any existing medical condition is under the best possible control e.g. diabetes, hypertension. This may require referral for appropriate advice.

b)   Any previous obstetric problems are fully assessed e.g. low birth weight baby.

c)   Any risk of hereditary disease is fully assessed. This may require referral to a clinical geneticist.

d)   The woman is as fit as possible prior to conceiving, for example:

immune to rubella
free from sexually transmitted disease
not smoking
minimal alcohol intake
good eating and exercise habits
not ingesting drugs

Investigations should provide a baseline to assess changes during pregnancy e.g. height, weight, blood pressure and breast and pelvic organs.

In order to ensure minimum standards of care the GP undertaking Maternity Medical Services is expected to provide care as outlined in Paragraph 31 Schedule 1 of the Statement of Fees and Advances (The Red Book). This states that a GP who has arranged to provide maternity medical services is responsible for providing all necessary medical services during pregnancy, confinement and the postnatal period, which includes the first 14 days after confinement and a full postnatal examination at or about 6 weeks after confinement. Obviously, if the woman is booked for hospital confinement the GPs obligations are reduced to the extent that the hospital takes responsibility for this time.

Paragraph 31 of Schedule 2 is concerned with the criteria for admission to the obstetric list. The obstetric list applicant has to satisfy the Local Obstetric Committee that he has sufficient experience; the minimum is usually a 6 month resident obstetric post. There are various options and consultation of the appropriate regulations is necessary to determine a person's eligibility. The GP who is on the obstetrics list can claim a higher fee for Maternity Medical Services.

Paragraph 31 of Schedule 3 describes good maternal and early neonatal care as might reasonably be expected to be provided by the GP providing maternity medical services. This paragraph has been reproduced from the 'Statement of Fees and Allowances (The Red Book)' with the permission of the Controller of Her Majesty's Stationery Office.

Memorandum on Maternal Care by General Practitioners

(Paragraph 31/Schedule 3)

Prepared on the advice of the Standing Maternity and Midwifery Advisory Committee and amended on the advice of the Standing Medical Advisory Committee and the Standing Nursing and Midwifery Advisory Committee.

1. The following note describes good maternal and early neonatal care such as might reasonably be expected under the maternity medical services. In undertaking to provide these services the general practitioner assumes responsibility for providing this standard of care. Normally he will be supported by attached midwives, health visitors and other members of the primary health care team.

First attendance
2. It will be necessary to confirm pregnancy and occasionally laboratory testing may be indicated. A detailed medical, obstetric, social and family history, followed by a careful examination are essential, for it is at this first attendance that the pattern of care the expectant mother is to receive should be mapped out.

3. The doctor will, of course, take into account any evidence of previous serious disease (e.g. cardiac, renal or respiratory) or accidents, including those diseases or accidents which may have resulted in a pelvic abnormality. Any complications occurring in or resulting from previous pregnancies affecting either the mother or child and any genetic condition must be considered. The progress of the present pregnancy to date, any risks arising from rubella, smoking habits, drug taking and any other factor which may affect the fetus should be checked. It is now well established that certain groups of women and their babies are particularly at risk from complications of pregnancy, labour and puerperium. These groups include primigravidae, multiparae over 35 years of age, mothers having their fourth or subsequent confinements, and women in social classes IV and V. The presence of any complicating factor or any such potential risk should suggest a referral for consultant advice so that the mother can have special care as early in the pregnancy as possible.

4.   Provisional arrangements should be made, usually at this stage, to book the mother's confinement in accordance with local obstetric policy; if she is to be delivered in an obstetric unit by someone other than her own doctor an early antenatal attendance there is desirable. It is not always possible to predict with complete certainty when complications may arise in any pregnancy and for this reason there are advantages for mothers to be delivered in an obstetric unit where full obstetric, paediatric and anaesthetic facilities are available. If, despite advice to the contrary, a mother insists on being confined at home, social factors in her case, including her accommodation, should be assessed by the primary health care team so that proper action can be taken later. Social factors also enter into decisions about postnatal transfer from hospital to home; any change in circumstances which would affect such a decision should be conveyed to the hospital concerned, so that premature transfer home is avoided.

5.   At the first attendance a record should be made of the mother's blood pressure, weight and the result of urine tests (which should if possible include a test for bacteriuria). Arrangements should always be made for blood to be taken, for the laboratory to estimate the haemoglobin, to group the mother's blood and to determine whether or not she is rhesus negative, to test for syphilis and to exclude in those groups of women at risk the presence of sickle cell disease or other abnormal haemoglobin. The need for chest X-ray should be considered in those women who are at medical or social risk of tuberculosis, particularly those from overseas areas where this condition is prevalent. When required it should preferably be performed between the 12th and 14th week of pregnancy and a full sized film should be used. Other X-ray examinations should normally be avoided. Ante-natal attendances present a good opportunity for taking a cervical smear, particularly from the high risk group. Arrangements should also be made for a dental examination. The fears and problems of many expectant mothers can often be discussed and allayed at this stage of pregnancy, so that at this and at all subsequent visits they should be encouraged to talk to the doctor and midwife. General advice should be given on diet, exercise, smoking and drug taking in pregnancy, and breast feeding, and an opportunity given them to discuss sexual or other difficulties. At this visit or later in pregnancy, when appropriate, a certificate of pregnancy (Form F W 8) should be completed. This form incorporates applications for exemption from prescription charges and where appropriate free milk tokens.

6.   Mothers benefit from ante-natal exercises, relaxation and parent-craft classes provided by the hospital or by community-based services and where such facilities are available the general practitioner should

consider the advantages to the mother in attending them. Fathers should also be encouraged to attend parent-craft classes.

7.   The utmost care should be taken over the prescribing of drugs in pregnancy, particularly in the first three months. The majority of doctors would advise the prescription of iron to pregnant women from the third month of pregnancy onwards; many would also advise a supplement of folic acid.

8.   Good record keeping with a system for readily identifying patients who fail to keep their appointments so that they can be followed up by the primary care team is an important factor of ante-natal care, particularly when care is shared with the hospital obstetric unit.

Subsequent examinations
9.   After the first examination, if the pregnancy proceeds normally, the patient should be seen at least once each month until the 28th week of pregnancy, at least fortnightly until the 34th to the 36th week and at least weekly thereafter, including the special examination at 30 to 34 weeks and at 36 weeks referred to in paragraphs 12 and 13 respectively. This is the routine suggested for a normal case; any suspicion of abnormality calls for more frequent supervision. (If possible such examinations should be carried out by the midwife and general practitioner together or a plan should be worked out to ensure that the expectant mother is seen by one or the other at these times.) Inconsistent advice to the mother can be avoided if there is a free interchange of information among the primary care team, by means of the co-operation card or by personal communication, between them and hospital staff if care is shared. When it is intended that the patient is to be delivered in a consultant obstetric unit the consultant will wish to see her at least once between the 34th and 36th week.

10.   At these examinations careful attention should be given to the mother's general health and nutrition, the abdomen should be examined, and a record made of blood pressure, weight and the results of urine tests; a further haemoglobin estimation should be made. The action to be taken on any evidence of abnormality is of course for decision by the general practitioner, but consultant advice should be sought in any case of doubt.

11.   The patient will need a certificate confirming pregnancy and the expected date of her confinement (Form Mat B1, or Form Mat B2, if the request for a certificate is made after the confinement has taken place) in order to enable her to claim any maternity benefits to which she may be entitled from her local Department of Health and Social Security Office.

Examination at 30 to 34 weeks

12.   Any obstetric abnormalities which are found will call for review of the plan for future care and full use should be made of consultant obstetric advice. Any slight rise in blood pressure, abnormal weight gain or loss, other evidence of pre-eclampsia or of the fetus being 'small for dates', should indicate the need for investigation or treatment. The haemoglobin estimation should be repeated at 30 weeks and treatment which has been given should be reviewed. In rhesus negative women a blood examination should also be carried out at 30 weeks for rhesus antibodies, and should these be detected, the patient will need to be referred for specialist advice. It is important that all cases in which the fetus appears to be small for the duration of gestation should be referred to a consultant for advice.

Examination at or about 36th week

13.   It is about this time that abnormalities likely to lead to difficult labour may be detected. Any suspicion of persistent malpresentation, disproportion, and other such conditions should lead to consultant obstetric advice being sought on the further management of the pregnancy. Where it is possible that the midwife may be required to initiate inhalational analgesia on her own responsibility, a certificate of the mother's fitness to receive it will be required beforehand.

14.   When labour does not occur within 10 days after the expected date of confinement this suggests that the advice of a consultant should be sought.

Care during labour

15.   If the mother is under the care of the general practitioner during labour it is clearly desirable that he should see the mother during labour, and it will be necessary for him to make suitable arrangements so that he is always available if summoned by the midwife. If he is not able to do so himself, he should arrange for a suitable experienced deputy to be available and should inform the midwife. Effective communication between the general practitioner and midwife is of paramount importance. In the light of the Report of the Confidential Enquiries into Maternal Deaths in England and Wales 1967–69, women receiving anaesthesia should, except in the most exceptional circumstances, receive care from a senior obstetrician and anaesthetist, and in the event of any serious complication with a home confinement the patient should be transferred to a fully equipped district hospital maternity unit or maternity hospital. In a major emergency in the patient's home or an isolated hospital unit the Emergency Obstetric Service (Obstetric Flying

Squad) can be called upon directly by the midwife if the doctor is not present and the delay in reaching him might endanger the patient's life.

Care of the newborn baby
16.   At the delivery, wherever the baby is born, there should be a recognised procedure for resuscitation, so that respiratory difficulties may be overcome before hypoxia can cause damage to the baby. It is essential therefore for the attendants including the general practitioner to be familiar with modern resuscitative techniques and they should normally have available an infant laryngoscope, endo-tracheal tubes, a bag to inflate and a mucus extractor.

17.   The immediate post-natal care of every infant, wherever it is born, should include a full clinical examination by a doctor trained and experienced in the detection of deviations from normal development. Apart from the immediate examination of the newborn it is the duty of the doctor to ensure that a complete clinical examination is made at about the 7th day. Local arrangements to test for phenylketonuria should be observed.

Puerperium
18.   Under the maternity medical services the general practitioner provides medical care for the mother and child for a period of 14 days after delivery. He should satisfy himself of the progress of the mother and child towards normal health and full rehabilitation and the establishment of a good mother/baby relationship. Advice on breast feeding should have been given during the antenatal period and encouragement should be continued.

19.   If the mother is rhesus negative the rhesus blood group of the baby should be determined. All rhesus negative women who have borne rhesus positive children and who have not been previously sensitised to the rhesus factor should be given anti-D-immunoglobulin as soon as possible and in any case no later than 60 hours after the birth of the child. (Haemolytic Disease of the Newborn October 1976 SMAC).

20.   All women should, at a time when they are receptive to it, have advice on family planning methods suitable to their case, genetic counselling, and if appropriate, sterilisation.

Post-natal examination
21.   At about six weeks after delivery, but not later than 12 weeks, the doctor should perform a medical examination of the mother. This would include examination of the genital tract. A cervical smear may be taken

where this has not been done in the ante-natal period. The subject of family planning may once more be raised. Arrangements for genetic counselling, if indicated, should also be made (Human Genetics July 1972 SMAC).

Miscarriage
22.   The general practitioner is often the only person in a key position to ensure that anti-D-immunoglobulin is given to all rhesus negative women following abortions, especially those who have had spontaneous abortions (Haemolytic Disease of the Newborn October 1976 SMAC).

3. THE MIDWIFE

Definition: "A midwife is a person who having been regularly admitted to a midwifery educational programme, duly recognised in the country in which it is located, has successfully completed the prescribed course of studies in midwifery and has acquired the requisite qualifications to be registered and/or legally licensed to practice midwifery.

Role: The midwife must be able to give necessary supervision, care and advice to women during pregnancy, labour and the postpartum period, to conduct deliveries on her own responsibility and to care for the newborn and infant. This care includes preventative measures, the detection of abnormal conditions in mother and child, the procurement of medical assistance and the execution of emergency measures in the absence of medical help. She has an important task in health counselling and education, not only for patients but also with the family and the community. The work should involve antenatal education and preparation for parenthood and extends to certain areas of gynaecology, family planning and child care. She may practise in hospitals, clinics, health units, domiciliary conditions or in any other service."

Activities: The activities of a midwife are defined in the European Community Midwives Directive.

1. To provide sound family planning information and advice.

2. To diagnose pregnancies and monitor normal pregnancies; to carry out examinations necessary for the monitoring of the development of normal pregnancies.

3. To prescribe or advise on the examinations necessary for the earliest possible diagnosis of pregnancies at risk.

4. To provide a programme of parenthood preparation and a complete preparation for childbirth including advice on hygiene and nutrition.

5. To care for and assist the mother during labour and to monitor the condition of the fetus in utero by the appropriate clinical and technical means.

6. To conduct spontaneous deliveries including where required an episiotomy and in urgent cases a breech delivery.

7. To recognise the warning signs of abnormality in the mother or infant which necessitate referral to a doctor and to assist the latter where appropriate; to take the necessary emergency measures in the doctor's absence, in particular the manual removal of the placenta, possibly followed by manual examination of the uterus.

8. To examine and care for the newborn infant; to take all initiatives which are necessary in case of need and to carry out where necessary immediate resuscitation.

9. To care for and monitor the progress of the mother in the post-natal period and to give all necessary advice to the mother on infant care to enable her to ensure the optimum progress of the newborn infant.

10. To carry out the treatment prescribed by a doctor.

11. To maintain all necessary records.

Supervision of practising midwives:

Present day maternity care is essentially the work of a team. Within this team the midwife has a defined sphere of practice and is accountable for her actions, professional judgement and the care she gives to mothers and babies.

The Nurses, Midwives and Health Visitors Act of 1979 makes provision for the supervision of midwives by Local Supervising Authorities. These include, the Regional Health Authority in England, the District Health Authority in Wales, the Health Boards in Scotland and the Social Services Boards in Northern Ireland. These local supervising Authorities may appoint 'Supervisors of Midwives'. Such persons are usually the senior midwifery managers within health authorities.

4. THE HEALTH VISITOR

Definition: "A health visitor is a state registered nurse who has undertaken a years full time study in preventative and social medicine and human development to obtain the health visitors certificate. She is often a state certified midwife and must possess an approved obstetric certificate".

Role: The health visitor has a large number of potential roles together with some statutory duties.

1. Post-natal home visiting. This is a statutory duty from the day the midwife stops attending (usually on the tenth day). The follow up usually continues until the child attends school. Their aim is to provide support and advice for the family during these early stages of parenthood. They should be able to recognise common postnatal problems and childhood illnesses making appropriate referrals to a doctor.

2. Child developmental and surveillance work. They should have a knowledge of the developmental milestones. Screening work is undertaken in the home and at child health clinics.

3. Preventative work + health education; this includes:

    Immunizations
    Health education for the local population
    Family planning advice
    Elderly population – visiting
          – screening
    This latter role is expanding as the elderly population grows. There is a new breed of health visitor with special interests in the elderly.

4. Liaison work.

    Knowledge of local resources
    Liaison with other health care professionals
    including the GP and social worker

5. Case work.

    Surveillance and support of at risk groups.

Supervision of Health Visitors:

Health visitors perform their duties as part of a team. Indeed approximately 90% are attached to practices. They are, however, employed by the District Health Authority and as such are accountable to the nursing managers within the health authority.

5. MATERNITY BENEFITS

This is often a confusing area for both the pregnant woman and health care professionals. It is important that those involved in providing care for the pregnant woman have sufficient knowledge of the benefits available to her. Up to date information can be obtained from the 'Hospital Welfare Rights Officer' based at the local social services department. The following is a summary of what is presently on offer.

A: WEEKLY MONEY

1. STATUTORY MATERNITY PAY

    This can be claimed if the pregnant woman is working or has worked recently. It is paid by employers if by the 26th week of pregnancy the woman has been working for them for at least six months and has paid national insurance contributions.

    Statutory maternity pay is paid weekly for 18 weeks. This can be taken to suit the pregnant woman but cannot be claimed before the 26th week of pregnancy and she must generally finish work no later than 6 weeks before the birth.

    If the woman has worked for the same employer for 2 years (full time) or 5 years (part time) by the time she is 26 weeks' gestation, then she is entitled to statutory maternity pay paid at 90% of the normal gross wage for the first six weeks. This then declines to the normal maternity pay which is currently £34.25 per week.

    The health care professionals need to provide the pregnant woman with a completed Mat B1 certificate so that she can claim statutory maternity pay. This form should be completed by the doctor or midwife no earlier than the 26th week of pregnancy and the expected date of confinement is noted.

2. MATERNITY ALLOWANCE

    This is paid to those who for some reason don't qualify for statutory maternity pay. The woman is entitled to this insurance if by the 26th week of pregnancy she has paid full national allowance contributions for six months out of the last year.

    It is currently £31.30 per week and is paid for 18 weeks consecutively. She needs to apply for this on the MA1 form from the DHSS.

3.   CHILD BENEFIT

As soon as the baby is born and the birth is registered then the woman can claim child benefit which is currently £7.25 per week. Single parent families can claim 'One Parent Benefit' on top of this. Again the DHSS has the claim forms.

4.   INCOME SUPPORT

This is paid to single women bringing up children alone. The amount paid varies with the woman's age. In addition to the weekly amount, help is given with mortgage interest, rent and rates. Income support also entitles the woman to milk tokens.

5.   FAMILY CREDIT

This has replaced Family Income Support (FIS) and is paid weekly to families on low wages.

B. LUMP SUMS

1.   MATERNITY PAYMENT

This can be claimed if the woman gets income support or family credit. It is designed as a payment towards maternity equipment. The woman can claim it at any time from the 30th week of pregnancy until the baby is 12 weeks old. It is currently a lump sum of £85 and the form (SF100) is available from the DHSS.

2.   SOCIAL FUND

This can be claimed if the woman gets income support. Usually payments are given on a LOAN basis and repayments are deducted from the weekly benefit. They are designed to pay for certain essential items such as clothing, furniture, cooker etc.

3.   HELP WITH TRAVEL COSTS

If the woman claims income support or family credit she can get a refund of travel costs for stays in hospital or antenatal appointments. Escorts can be claimed for if medically needed. These are claimed from the hospital general office.

6. USEFUL DEFINITIONS AND DIFFICULT EXAM TOPICS

1. Fetal distress

This is a clinical condition in which the utero-placental unit fails to provide adequate oxygenation or nutrition to the fetus. It may occur antenatally or intrapartum.

Antenatal fetal distress may be acute or chronic.

The acute causes are from cord accidents, prolapse or presentation, or abruptio-placentae. Acute placental failure may occur in diabetic pregnancy, resulting in still birth. The chronic causes are mainly concerned with intra-uterine growth retardation, such as hypertensive cases, heavy smokers and alcohol abusers. In certain cases acute fetal distress may occur on chronic e.g. accidental haemorrhage in a growth retarded hypertensive case.

Intrapartum fetal distress.

This is defined as:

a. an abnormal fetal heart rate pattern
b. meconium stained amniotic fluid
c. pH less than 7.20.

Common causes of intrapartum fetal distress:

1. Uterine hyperstimulation – excessive use of oxytocics.
2. Cord problems – prolapsed cord, cord compression or cord knots.
3. Hypotension – epidural anaesthesia, dehydration due to prolonged labour.
4. Keto-acidosis.
5. 'Placental insufficiency – intrauterine growth retardation'.
6. Abruptio placentae.

It should be noted that the worst fetal heart rate pattern is a complicated fetal tachycardia. This occurs when the base rate is above 160 beats per minute and there are additional abnormalities in the trace such as decelerations or loss of beat to beat variation. In these cases fetal hypoxia occurs in 50–55%. To attain greater accuracy in interpretation of traces, a fetal scalp pH is required!

2. Vertex

This is the area on the fetal skull bounded by:

1. Coronal suture (anterior fontanelle).
2. Parietal eminences.
3. Lamboidal sutures (posterior fontanelle).

The vertex is part of the fetal head which negotiates the birth canal when there is flexion and the denominator is the occiput.

3. Asynclitism

This is the phenomenon by which the fetal head negotiates the pelvic inlet in a 'rocking' fashion whereby one parietal bone leads the other (occipito-transverse position). If the anterior parietal bone leads then the term is anterior asynclitism. This is of practical importance when rotational forceps are required to rotate a malposition. The sliding lock in Kiellands forceps allows for asynclitism to be corrected.

4. The Lower Segment

This is the lower aspect of the uterus *below* the utero-vesical reflection of peritoneum. It corresponds to the isthmus in the non-pregnant uterus. The lower segment starts to form from approximately 26 weeks' gestation but is not properly formed until after 32 weeks. This is of practical importance when performing caesarean sections. The presence of placental tissue in the lower segment constitutes the condition of placenta praevia to either minor or major degrees.

The lower segment has less muscle fibre and contains more fibrous connective tissue than the upper segment. The scar in the lower segment caesarean section thus heals strongly and is less likely to rupture in a subsequent labour unlike that in the upper segment (classical) scar.

The lower segment is located within 3 ins [7.5 cm] of the internal os.

5. Engagement

This is when the widest part of the fetal skull (BPD) has negotiated the pelvic inlet. In practice, this means that two-fiths of the head, or less, is palpable on abdominal examination. On vaginal examination the head would therefore be at the level of the ischial spines.

Difficult Exam Topics

1. Surgery in gynaecological malignancy

The basic operation for the treatment of carcinoma of the pelvic viscera is *Total hysterectomy and bi-lateral salpingo-oophorectomy* (TAH + BSO).

It should be noted that the excision of an enlarged ovary is known as an *ovariectomy,* whereas excision of a normal sized ovary is *oophorectomy.*

The site of the primary carcinoma determines any additional surgery to the TAH + BSO. To rationalise the need for additional surgery it is necessary to have some knowledge of the nature of the specific disease:

1) **Carcinoma of the cervix:** This tumour which tends to be mainly squamous carcinoma spreads readily to the *lymphatics* and by *local* invasion to the parametria and upper vagina. It is, therefore, essential to perform pelvic lymphadenectomy, excision of parametria and upper third of vagina. This constitutes what is known as the extended hysterectomy or Wertheim's hysterectomy. In young women the ovaries are often conserved. Squamous carcinoma is *radio sensitive,* and therefore the treatment of choice is usually radiotherapy in the older age groups.

2) **Endometrial carcinoma:** Carcinoma of the endometrium spreads less readily to the lymphatics, except when local invasion of the myometrium extends to the outer third or serosa. A common site for secondary spread is the upper vagina and ovaries, hence in addition to the hysterectomy + BSO, a cuff of vagina is excised.

3) **Ovary:** Except for the disgerminoma, cancers of the ovary are radio *insensitive.* The mainstay of treatment, therefore, is surgical supported by chemotherapy. Carcinoma of the ovary spreads in a classic transcoelomic manner, producing studding or deposits over the peritoneal cavity associated with ascites. The tumour is, therefore, commonly located in the omentum and other ovary.

Hence omentectomy and both ovaries are commonly excised. The removal of the uterus in carcinoma of the ovary is a little contentious, but it is better removed as there can be associated neoplastic change in the endometrium. Peritoneal washings at laparotomy may also show malignant cells on cytological examination when there is no obvious clinical evidence of metastases.

4) **Fallopian tube:** This is a rare tumour and tends to be similar in behaviour to endometrium and cancers of the ovary. Therefore, total hysterectomy and BSO is often sufficient supported with post-operative chemotherapy.

The understanding of the nature of these carcinomas will enable you to answer questions more readily on the treatment of these conditions.

Once again, the basic operation for removal of carcinoma of the pelvic viscera is *total hysterectomy and bi-lateral salpingo-oophorectomy.*

2. Discuss the principles of drug therapy in the treatment of endometriosis.

Answer:

Endometriosis is the condition in which there is ectopic or misplaced endometrial-like tissue outside the uterine cavity. This misplaced tissue is responsive to cyclical hormones, hence it bleeds at menstrual times and mainly produces symptoms related to menstruation; dysmenorrhoea and menorrhagia. The subsequent inflammatory reaction in the pelvis leads to chronic pelvic pain, dyspareunia and subfertility.

The treatment entails:

1. abolition of menstruation or
2. creating a pseudo pregnancy state.

1. Abolition of menstruation

This can be achieved by using an anti-gonadotrophin agent, danazol. The side effects include nausea and vomiting, fluid retention, weight gain, cramps and mild masculinisation. It is not surprising that compliance with the therapy is poor. Another agent is an LH/RH analogue which may be administered intra-nasally or by injections. Reports suggest there are fewer side effects and this may well be effective treatment in the future.

2. Pseudo pregnancy

This is achieved by using progestogens. It is important to emphasise that the treatment should be *continuous* and *not* cyclical. Breakthrough bleeding is commonly encountered, but usually overcome by increasing the dosage.

The duration of the above therapies relates to the extent of the disease.

It is usual for patients with severe endometriosis to be on therapy for at least twelve months; six to eight months with mild endometriosis. If there is any doubt about discontinuation of therapy, then repeat laparoscopy is necessary.

3. Describe the intrapartum care of a breech presentation.

Answer:

This is a contentious subject and obstetricians differ greatly in their views. A 'middle of the road approach' therefore needs to be adopted. Assuming there have been no antenatal complications, maternal pelvis is adequate and the fetal weight average (2.5–3.5 kg), the patient should be delivered in a *Consultant Unit*. There should be adequate anaesthetic and paediatric facilities, together with a theatre for emergency Caesarean section.

The labour should be managed by an experienced obstetrician and midwife supported by similarly experienced anaesthetist and paediatrician.

The risks in breech labour are mainly due to the fetus; hypoxia and trauma. The dangers are minimised by the following management.

First Stage

1.   Continuous fetal heart rate monitoring.
2.   Epidural analgesia (avoids narcotics, provides analgesia, prevents premature pushing, and facilitates forceps to the after coming head).

3.   If problems, early resort to Caesarean section.

Second Stage – assisted breech delivery

This technique is based on expulsion of the fetus by maternal effort and uterine contractions. Minimal handling by the obstetrician is mandatory.

The patient is put in the lithotomy position when the anterior fetal buttock is visible. With maternal effort in phase with uterine contractions, the buttocks, legs and trunk are delivered. At this point it is permissible for the obstetrician to gently hold the baby over the posterior iliac crests, thus avoiding trauma to the abdominal viscera. Further maternal effort should facilitate the delivery of the arms. Extended arms may require the use of Loveset's manoeuvres. When the baby is delivered to the nape of its neck, it should be carefully extended towards the maternal abdomen. The obstetrics forceps (Wrigley's or Simpson's) should then be applied and the head delivered at a controlled rate to avoid a precipitate delivery resulting in intra-cranial haemorrhage or conversely a slow delivery which would result in cerebral hypoxia. The value of epidural analgesia, in assisted breech deliveries, cannot be over emphasised. It should be equally stressed that at any time during the first or second stages of labour there are signs of fetal distress or delay in labour or descent of the breech, Caesarean section should be performed.

4.   What does Syntometrine consist of and how does it work?

Answer:

Syntometrine consists of 5 units of syntocinon and 0.5 mg ergometrine. It is usually administered intra-muscularly at delivery of the anterior shoulder. The syntocinon stimulates a uterine contraction approximately 2 minutes later. The contraction is sustained by the tetanic action of the ergometrine which takes effect after 7 minutes. The resultant effect of these two agents is that the uterus is stimulated rapidly and maintained in a contracted state to facilitate delivery of the placenta and reduce the risk of post partum haemorrhage.

The vasoconstrictive properties of ergometrine make the drug contra-indicated in cardiac cases, hypertensive and pre-eclamptic patients. In such cases syntocinon is used in preference.

REVISION INDEX